MAN HEAL THYSELF

JOURNEY TO OPTIMAL WELLNESS

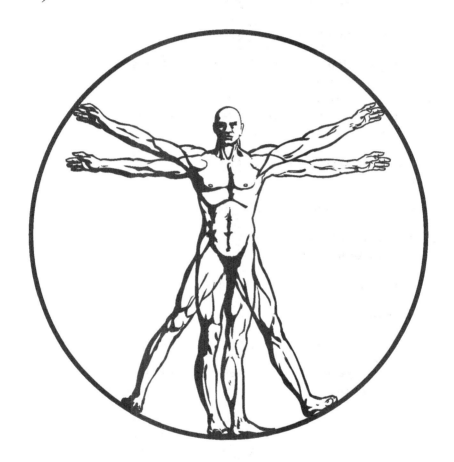

BY QUEEN AFUA

Man Heal Thyself: Journey to Optimal Wellness
Publishing 2012 by Afrikan World Books

By Queen Afua/Helen O. Robinson

Library of Congress Cataloging in Publication Data
Queen Afua.

Illustrations: Rafael Montalvo, montalvodesigns@gmail.com

Cover Art and Design: Rafael Montalvo, www.montalvodesigns.com
montalvodesigns@gmail.com

Text Design & Layout: Cindy Shaw, CreativeDetails.net

Developmental Editor: Gerianne F. Scott

Assistant Editor: Dawn Walton

Typists: De'Arcy Ba-Ra Livingston; Sacred Women: Tabia Beckett, Nivia Golson, Tonyia Madison, Tacarra Moore, Terri Murray, Andrea Spencer, Tarshay Williams

Published by Afrikan World Books
POB 16447, Baltimore, MD 21217
tel: 410-383-2006
www.afrikanworldbooks.com

"MAY I OPEN MY TWO EYES
WHICH ARE BLIND.

MAY I STRETCH OUT MY FEET
WHICH ARE FASTENED TOGETHER.

MAY MY LEGS BE STRONG AND RAISE ME UP.

I KNOW MY HEART,

I HAVE GAINED POWER OVER
MY HANDS AND ARMS.

I HAVE GAINED POWER OVER
MY TWO FEET.

I HAVE GAINED THE POWER TO DO
WHAT PLEASETH MY SOUL.

MAY MY SOUL AND BODY
NOT BE IMPRISONED.

I RISE AND SHINE…

I AM POWERFUL, I AM MIGHTY,

I COME FORTH IN PEACE."

FROM THE PAPYRUS OF ANI
(TRANSLITERATION AND TRANSLATION BY E.A. WALLIS BUDGE)

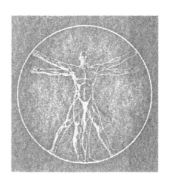

CONTENTS

DEDICATION

I dedicate Man Heal Thyself: Journey To Optimal Wellness to the million men who created the historical Million Man March in Washington D.C. on October 16, 1995. As the world, watched you travelled by bus, by plane, by train and on foot to unite in oneness for atonement. May you always be a vision of that unity; a symbol of transformation, of healing, of love and of power. May you continue to RISE UP, overcome, align, and step forward. I offer this document to you men, each on his quest to Heal Thyself.

Men, who are in pain and in need of healing, I dedicate Man Heal Thyself to you.

Men, who were abused and, so, have become abusers, as you search for change and transformation I dedicate Man Heal Thyself to you.

Men, starving for peace of mind, wholeness, fulfillment and encouragement; I dedicate Man Heal Thyself to you.

Men, with broken hearts, smashed limbs, shattered dreams and worn souls; I dedicate Man Heal Thyself to you.

Young men, of the up and coming generation, I dedicate Man Heal Thyself to you. May you walk well and walk strong throughout your journey to optimal wellness.

I dedicate Man Heal Thyself to you men who find fulfillment, strength, and refuge in your healing -- those who keep on keeping on; but especially to you who have lost your way in life's maze.

I dedicate Man Heal Thyself to you men who are enjoying the freedom of not being incarcerated; but especially to you who are incarcerated.

Men, who are enjoying wellness which includes financial wealth and stability; I dedicate, Man Heal Thyself to continued success on your wellness journey.

To the millions of men in the United States and globally who are uninsured, unprotected, uncared for, unloved and left for dead; I humbly dedicate Man Heal Thyself to you. May you gain support, momentum and strength to pursue your wellness.

Finally, I dedicate Man Heal Thyself to all of the mothers, grandmothers, wives, sisters and lovers, who stand... wait...and pray, as the men travel on their journeys to heal themselves.

WHAT IS TIME? WHAT TIME IS IT?

As an AstroNumerologist, time means everything to me. First of all, time is of the essence! Now, you can take your sweet time if you want to, but time moves with precision and waits for no one. Time is a measure of things. Time is a guide of how long one has to do things and how much gets done. Imagine, for example, telling a woman baking bread in the oven that she can come back to check on it "anytime" she wishes, let's say, next week or next month? With that miscalculation of the time needed to do the task it would be a wonder if she came back in a week and still had an oven left in the kitchen, much less the bread.

But we do not have to imagine appropriate or inappropriate uses of time. We can and must focus on what time is it now. It is time to get things done in a quick and orderly manner. Most importantly, it is time that every man—young and old—pick up a copy of Queen Afua's amazing book, *Man Heal Thyself: Journey to Optimal Wellness*. It is time that we men act on the truth and the power to be found within the pages of this book. Men, we must begin the process of moving from "Wounded Man to Supreme Man Optimal Wellness."

It has always been a given that Queen Afua's role, among many, is to empower women, especially with regard to their health. That comes as no surprise if you've ever had the pleasure of meeting this wonder spirit. Her smile is like the sun, the symbol of her zodiac sign, Leo. More importantly, being around her aura or presence is healing in itself. When you can't help but return a smile you end up listening to what she is talking about. And, many have been listening. Over the years I have personally observed how the health of clients of mine had improved once they began eating naturally and organically as Queen suggests. Now, men, it is time for us to begin to pay attention to our healing. As you get into this jewel of a book, it's obvious that Queen Afua is very aware of the male species and our way of thinking, acting and Being. Queen Afua's *Man Heal Thyself: Journey to Optimal Wellness* provides checklists to get us up to speed and keep us on track. Step-by-step, she guides us to raise our awareness, heighten our consciousness and understand the true role healthy living habits play on our state of being.

What is required of us men is to own up to the myths and misplaced motives we have about ourselves and our relationships. It is time to take responsibility for our behavior, which eventually has an impact not only on our lives but also on the women and children in our lives. *Man Heal Thyself* should be shared with the younger generation to guide them to become better individuals. To delay reading this book or to delay beginning the processes outlined in this book would be unwise. The last thing we need to do is waste our precious time. Men, we need to be where we men need to be; and we need to get on time about it. The value of reading and working through this guide to personal growth and development is priceless. Learning to actually transform yourself and your life in ways that you haven't experienced in years, or maybe ever, should be enough to motivate any man. Wow...just the thought of it staggers the imagination!

It is time.

LLoyd Strayhorn

LLoyd Strayhorn, World Renowned AstroNumerologist/Author of The best seller: *Numbers and You*
Coming in 2012 -2013: Lloyd's Book of Numbers A numerology guide for the 21st Century
numbersandyou.com /1 800 581 4401

FOREWORD 2

TIME TO RECALIBRATE

I am remembering… I give thanks to the women who played significant roles in reflecting to me my consciousness; to the women who tolerated my egotistical approach to life and still managed to love me through it all. To discount those relationships as "failures" would be a disregard of their perfection reflection.

The call of **MAN HEAL THYSELF** is a resounding call for support, accountability and responsibility. The same call is demonstrated in the Olmec-Mayan Prophesy of 2012, where Time's Special Witness, Pacal Votan, the Mayan Prophet's tomb was discovered deep within the Pyramid of The Inscriptions on June 15, 1952 in Palenque, Mexico. The return of the feminine is illustrated in the hieroglyphs within the Pyramid, and revealed to us through the work of Natural Time scholar, Valum Votan (aka The Closer of the Cycle, aka Jose Arguelles) in this quote from *Living Through the Closing of the Cycle—A Survival Guide for the Road to 2012:*

> "Until the discovery of the tomb of the Red Queen on June 1, 1994, Pascal's tomb was considered unique, but the tomb of the Red Queen …was a further clue. Identical to that of Pacal, the tomb of the Red Queen also featured a jade mask and a speaking tube. The only difference between the two tombs is that the tomb of Pacal Votan is laden with inscription, while that of the Red Queen has none. These two tombs are … intentionally placed to be a sign for us in the end times…"

And further:

"Our tombs are side by side. The one in the Temple of the Inscriptions contains all the clues both of your Earth history as well as of the cosmic history. It is in the Temple of the Inscriptions, because what is written or inscribed refers to the original book, the Mother of the Book. That is the conscious side of cosmic history. This is the tomb of the man for it is the men who 'made' history. But now your little history is over. That is the meaning of 2012. That is also the meaning of the other tomb, that of the Red Queen, the woman, the one oppressed by history. That is why this tomb is devoid of inscriptions. It represents the unconscious side of cosmic history now waking up in the Closing of the Cycle. It is in Temple XIII because the harmonic salvation of your race and your planet lies in the calendar cycle of thirteen moons. She whose tomb this is, we call the Red Queen."

The prophesy of Pacal Votan is known as the Telektonon or Earth Spirit Speaking Tube. This prophesy was revealed in the same year that the tomb of the Red Queen was discovered and declares that the only way to make it to 2012 in harmony is by changing the calendar. We can all be on the 2013 Red Road of feminine resurrection after the long-awaited end-cycle of the Black Road—2012. The 300 year period of the infamous "1712 Willie Lynch Papers" has us at the crossroads and it is leading us to restore the LAW of MAÁT). This immutable law gives us the true time frequency of 13:20 (a paradigm of time measurement based on the feminine anatomy and the feminine frequency of existence.) It is the recalibration of our Cosmic Time Travel through our Galactic Purpose Signature (GPS) in order to navigate Time Ship Earth into 2013 recounting the Lover's Script of Pacal Voton and Bolon Ik. (The newest information from José Argüelles (aka Valum Votan) and Lloydine Argüelles (aka Bolon Ik) is *The 20 Tablets of the Law of Time*).

We are coming full circle and we—both man and woman must HEAL ourselves to navigate safely into the new paradigm. Whether or not we continue the conversation begun here regarding the recalibration of how we measure time, we must adjust to the way we use our time to attain our wellness. Most women have begun this recalibration. Men, we must begin to do the same. Queen Afua's call to action is a one-stop service station designed to tune-up

our temporary space suits so we can continue on our journey into the new paradigm of light and love. Our ancestors beseech us to, "heed to the call y'all," and we will arise gracefully from our fall. MAN, recalibrate and heal thyself.Asante Sana! Tua Neter! Medase!
Wanique Khemi Tehuti Shabazz

Wanique Khemi Tehuti Shabazz/Director of Operations, WRFG 89.3 FM, Atlanta / www.wrfg.org
On "Time Travel": www.waniqueshabazz.com and www.melanin6.com.

References and Excerpts from Jose Arguelles author of *"Time, Synchronicity, and Calendar Change; Living Through the Closing of the Cycle, A Survival Guide for the Road to 2012* / website: www.lawoftime,org.

FOREWORD 3

"Queen made me aware that I could heal myself...she was the first
to talk to me about life with the solution being life."
-NOREAGA, HIP HOP ARTIST

TIME TO RESTORE

I cannot express the appreciation that I have to my mother for writing a wellness book for men, about men, and in honor of men. My holistic wellness training about what to eat and how to take care of my body began from birth. As a child, my mother had me teach and conduct workshops in yoga and Tai-Chi to her client's children. Later, when I was a teenager, my mother asked me to give words of encouragement to her teenage clients while she consulted with their parents. We were a mother-son wellness team. I was honored! So it made sense that when I became a young man, my mother asked me, to continue to address my peers, who had become known as 'Generation X'. I spoke to young men - our future - about their wellness future. I told them, "Wake up and be healed!"

I wrote *The Remedy*. This is a call to my community and the new generation at large: WAKE UP!!! IT IS A STATE OF EMERGENCY, AND WE ARE IN AN URGENT HEALTH CRISIS! OUR FAMILIES ARE DYING. MY GENERATION OF MEN IS THE FIRST THAT MAY NOT OUT LIVE THEIR PARENTS!!

As we mourn the passing of hip-hop icon, Guru, I challenge all of his peers and fans to not let his death be in vain. There is no reason that Guru and so many others under forty-five years old should be passing away at the rate they are. Every MC, B-Boy, DJ, Graf Artist, college student, "brutha" on the corner, G, and hustler is personally suffering from or knows someone battling cancer, arthritis, diabetes, asthma, hypertension, obesity, and many other ill-nesses. Most of these illnesses are caused or worsened by the foods we eat.

Don't think for one minute your aunties, big mamas, and parents are the only ones battling these sicknesses. African-American and Latino communi-ties lead the statistics for all of these crippling diseases, and people under age forty are being hit at alarming rates. According to the Office of Minority Health, about one in four African-American women are overweight or obese and nearly 20% of African-American children are at high risk for blood pres-sure, diabetes, high cholesterol, and a slew of other obesity-related diseases.

It is the fast food and over-processed, pre-packaged US food culture that has driven us to this place; and if we do not act soon, we may not be able to turn back. You still think this does not apply to you? Or perhaps you just need some extra reinforcement. Read the list below of globally renowned male celebrities who have battled major life-threatening health conditions. This list represents sons, and fathers, and the men of this generation; the men of our future.

MC Breed:	Dead at 37 – Kidney Failure
J. Dilla:	Dead at 32 – Cardiac Arrest
Big Pun:	Dead at 28 – Heart Attack
Nate Dogg:	Dead at 41 – Stroke
Alonzo Mourning, 40:	Kidney Disease; Kidney transplant at 33
Ghostface Killah, 39:	Diagnosed with Type 1 Diabetes at 26
Lil Boosie, 27:	Diagnosed with type 1 Diabetes at 26; Takes insulin 3 times a day
Phife Dawg, 39:	Type 1 Diabetes; has had a Kidney Transplant
Heavy D:	Dead at 44 -Stroke – Also, now, too soon an ancestor

This is only a short list of famous people who have disclosed their health status to the public. Even though these people do not lack money, they still fall sick with dis-ease because they lack the knowledge of how to "Heal Thyself." You don't have to be old, poor, overweight, or living in the hood to be sick. We suffer from lack of knowledge. This is a microcosmic list of what is taking place with our men on a macrocosmic level.

Beyond being a hip-hop artist, I am a second generation holistic health advocate. I have traveled the road with Grammy Award winner, hip hop singer, songwriter Erykah Badu as her wellness coach. Over the years I have encountered countless celebrities dealing with minor and major aliments. On the personal front, I am sick and tired of losing young people and reading depressing statistics. At this point NOBODY IS EXEMPT. Everyone is vulnerable to these diseases and unless we make some immediate major changes to in-corporate healthier eating habits and lifestyle practices, my generation might not live to see fifty years old. If you are living on the American diet YOU TOO ARE A WALKING, TICKING TIME BOMB ready to explode at any moment from the constant build up of fast food, fried foods, candy, sodas, sugar drinks, and chemical additives you are constantly ingesting. I am talking to YOU.

In her book *City of Wellness* Queen Afua writes about the fast food corporate kitchens. Most people know that this kind of food is bad for them, but they continue to eat this way every single day. So I ask everyone at what point are we going to WAKE UP?!!! The number one excuse people give for unhealthy eating is that eating healthy costs too much. Yet, many of these same people spend hundreds of dollars on expensive, so-called luxury sneak-ers, hand bags, car rims, and other material indulgences. When we tell these same people, who may buy two or three bottles in the club, to go buy a juicer, they say it is too expensive or they simply laugh it off. Our priorities are horribly messed up when it comes to spending money and taking care of ourselves. People care more about what they look like from the outside than they do about how their bodies are working on the inside. They are more concerned with being able to participate in the, 'Pass the... —Blame it on the Alcohol' lifestyle, than learning to do away with the sicknesses that force them to take medication daily. They would rather invest in expensive shoes than work to prevent diabetes that could one day lead to amputations and no options to wear shoes.

Big Pun passed, and we didn't take heed. Nate Dogg had two strokes and passed, and not much was said. When we lost J. Dilla people finally started to show some concern. When Phife Dawg exposed his battle with diabetes, people began to realize that there is an issue. Still, no one has effectively challenged our generation on a widespread scale to reclaim our wellness at every level.

I challenge the men to "Man Up" and "Heal Thyself" as my mother, Queen Afua, guides you on The Journey to Wellness. I challenge you to lead a lifestyle, not of dis-ease that will continue to disable you, but rather of wellness that will holistically empower your life as a Man.

Supa Nova Slom

Supa Nova Slom, Holistic Wellness Warrior, Hip Hop Medicine Author of:
The Remedy

FOREWORD 4

THOUGHTS FROM THE EXAMINATION ROOM

From the sacred space of the Doctor's Exam Room, where men and women surrender pretense and ego to the desire to find answers, avoid pain and prolong life, I join my voice with my fellow collaborators to repeat the timeliness of this work and the urgency of the situation.

I have been a practicing, traditionally trained licensed and Board Certified Family Practitioner for thirty years. My entire career has been spent in two zip codes in Brooklyn, New York. The observations that I have made during that time are, no doubt, reflected in many other places around the country—rural, urban, upper class, and inner city. As a nation, we are becoming technologically advanced, but these impressive strides do not reflect in a healthier population. In the 21st Century, people still succumb to the same chronic illness as three decades ago, and at much higher rates. Lack of access to care and information are minor reasons for the quantum leap to near epidemic numbers of Hypertension, Type 2 Diabetes, Heart Disease and Cancer. People fill the clinics and offices in record numbers. At the same time the Internet has made us all "research experts" and prescription drug sales account for billions of dollars in the Health Care Budget. Nonetheless the statistics do not redeem us as a healthier population.

The last, chilling piece of the equation, the one that frosts the cake of urgency, is the fact that the children are now joining the ranks of the chronically ill, succumbing to "adult diseases" before they are even old enough to vote.

We literally are dying to be well.

The solution, of course, is not found in a single place, but in a collaborative effort of things simple and things complex. There is no turning away from the fact that a toxic lifestyle based on consuming toxic food while growing up and growing old in a stressful century will require more and more pharmaceutical intervention to suppress its toxic effects. This book represents the first step to self-healing and the simple realization that the car runs better and breaks down less if you fill it with quality fuel. It provides a template for healing, clear thinking, forgiveness and release. Its message could not be timelier.

Kudos, thanks and professional respect to Queen Afua, whom I have the privilege to know as a colleague and friend. From our first encounter, we recognized each other as healers on a common road. Because of that recognition and mutual respect, we have been able to blend our knowledge for a common good, proving that, yes; it is possible for holistic strategies and mainstream medical to align. It is my hope and desire that her book finds a home in the consciousness of every man who reads it. To transform one, ultimately has an effect on all.

Respectfully submitted,
Bernadette L. Sheridan

Bernadette L. Sheridan MD, F.A.A.F.P
CEO, Grace Family Medical Practice /Brooklyn, NY

PREFACE

The Creator Has a Master Plan

"The Creator has a master plan, peace and happiness for every man.
The Creator has a working plan, peace and happiness for every man.
The Creator makes but one demand, happiness through all the land."
PHARAOH SANDERS/1969

THE MASTER PLAN

The late 1960s was a time of Freedom Fighting and "Power to the People; and the dawn of a Holistic Revolution. There were "black shops" in urban areas across the United States including in my neighborhood in Brooklyn, New York. The black shops appealed to all my senses. Inside there were cowry shells in wooden bowls and posters of Angela Davis and Malcolm X on the walls. I could touch imported earrings, try on colorful African dashikis and smell sweet frankincense, myrrh and cinnamon incense. Stereo speakers were posted outside the front doors so passersby could enjoy the "Black talk" and "Black music" of the times. The music of Pharaoh Saunders always lured me inside. Saunders' masterpiece was to become my mantra; the anthem that has shaped me through all the seasons of my life. "The Creator Has a Master Plan" …What was the plan that was going to liberate my people and people suffering globally to achieve "peace and happiness" and wholeness?

I was seventeen.

I began my quest to help others right after I had been forced to help myself, at least forty years ago. I had been suffering from so many illnesses the doctor had told my mother, "Your daughter is so sick she should live in a glass house." He said he could not help me. I had to help myself. The solution was within. For one season I fasted and detoxed and worked on healing holistic myself. Eventually I was rid of chronic asthma, arthritis, eczema, headaches and depression. The techniques of detoxification and purification were working. I studied them further, enough to become certified as a holistic health consultant and a colon therapist. In order to help others I opened a wellness center on Flatbush Avenue in Brooklyn, New York. Although I was guiding thousands through the 21 Day Fasting Program I had developed, I was still seeking to find the Master Plan that was going to liberate people to achieve "peace and happiness" and wellness. As I continued studying our history, I learned that the plan I was looking for had been written as the Principle of Maát in the ancient temples of the Ancient Ones (The Shining Beings of my Ancestors). The writings describe how to Heal Thyself in order to live in optimal balance, wellness and righteousness. I learned that achieving the Master Plan is an attainable goal. I wrote the little green book *Heal Thyself for Health & Longevity* and traveled beyond Brooklyn to share what I had learned.

In my travels around the world men asked, "What about me, Queen? You keep speaking about the women, but what about the men?" My response was, "In order to Heal Thyself, you have to show up, step forward, stand up, activate, fight for and follow through for your healing. Actually, the women folk have been waiting for you. We have gathered in circles of Sisters to help each other overcome our pain and we've been hoping you would join us and start looking out for yourselves." I had written *Heal Thyself* for the whole family, but it was mostly the women who had been showing up for consultations, wellness workshops, Fasting Shut–Ins, Detox Seminars and colonic irrigations. I had not seen the men stepping up for their wellness in large numbers.

Since mostly women were listening I continued speaking to them and went on to write *Sacred Woman: A Guide to Healing the Feminine Body, Mind & Spirit*. The women continued responding to the task of restoration and rejuvenation. We continued to watch and wait for the men to respond. Some men came with female family members, but again, not in large numbers. I made *another* attempt to reach out to you; I even the put the Wellness Man on the cover of *The City of Wellness: Restoring Your Health Through the Seven Kitchens of Consciousness*. Still, over the next 4 years, the men I saw were few and far between. The women were working on their wellness and many went from being concerned to being angry that the men were not doing their part to become well. I addressed the cause and remedy for this anger in my next book, *Overcoming an Angry Vagina: Journey to Womb Wellness*. At last, the men started calling me in larger numbers. "What about me?" The women echoed, "What about the men, Queen?" I reminded the women that they were the primary healers of the family in the home. I told them to follow the teachings of the Ancient Ones:

September 2010, I was nearly drowned in a catastrophic shift in my personal and professional life. My business and I were in need of refuge which my CEO and son, Ali, reached out for and obtained for us. Fredrica Bey, assisted by her daughter, Amenia, became my guardian angel. With the approval of the Board of Directors of Wisommm (Women In Support of the Million Man March, Inc.) I was offered a place to house myself and my work until I could get on my feet. I lived and worked in the Wisommm Cultural Center on the 5th floor of a building that also housed a massive cathedral. Every night at 10:00 PM the doors were locked and the safety alarm was activated. My vision, my boxes and I were locked in all night! At 6:00 in the morning the alarm was turned off and school was re-opened on the lower level. For five months I had time to reflect on my next steps as a wellness advocate. Throughout this "test", I carried on business as usual; I consulted, gave workshops and prepared and distributed my formulas, internationally. Oh, yes, it was challenging and even overwhelming sometimes. But I kept reminding myself…'*The Creator has a Master Plan'*.

"I am the woman who lightens the darkness. I have come to lighten the darkness. It is lightened…"

At 9:00 PM, one night, during my fourth month in the monastery of Wisommm, I heard a rumbling from under my floor. What must have been hundreds of men from the Nation of Islam were chanting! It sounded like they were raising the roof; and it felt like the powerful stomping of a Zulu tribal dance. The men were anticipating the arrival of the Honorable Minister Luis Farrakhan, but he had been delayed at the United Nations and was not able to come to The Wisommm Cultural Center. Nonetheless, the men's enthusiastic chanting had surely opened the gates within me to take on my work; to answer the call. That night I was given yet one more sign to write this book, *Man Heal Thyself*.

The final and perhaps most outstanding sign to write the book also took place at the Wisommm Center. On a Friday night the doors were opened to community activists, the media, the police department, and parents whose children had been murdered and other concerned citizens of New Jersey. It seemed like thousands had shown up for a rally focused on stopping the violence and saving our community from any more blood-shed. I was there in the midst of it all and I was praying for our healing. The next night after sunset, I had just finished teaching an Emerald Green Practitioner Training when the lights suddenly went out. I tried everything to get them back on, and at the time there was no one in the building. I did not know what to do. I had to prepare for the next day of wellness work and the pressure was on. So I asked the Most High, "What am I going to do in the dark?" I heard from within, "Light a candle and write." So I lit a candle, and burned incense and for seven hours I channeled the beginnings of *Man, Heal Thyself.* No distractions, just a candle, a light in my heart, and a vision whose time had come!

Slowly I began to write *Man Heal Thyself.* It was difficult. I kept on writing until I decided to create a scroll. In ninety hours I wrote two scrolls, "Man Heal Thyself Scroll 1 & 2". "Done" I thought to myself, "Maybe, now I *don't* need to write the book; I said it all on the scrolls!" I used the completed scrolls to conduct the first Man Heal Thyself training workshop to three brave souls who were vested in healing themselves. In the midst of the workshop one of the participants said, "Queen, you might as well write a book." "Who asked him?" I thought to myself. But I already knew what time it was. I'm born on the 13th. Four is my number, and this is a four year for me, and the

Heal Thyself training is based on the 4 elements. All the signs are in place. I accept fully. No longer is writing this book hard. It is a joy, an honor; and it is part of the Master Plan.

'I am the woman who lightens the darkness; I have come to lighten the darkness, it is lightened.'

The Master Plan is Healing Thyself. It is an ongoing miracle. I humbly share that according to plan I am on the path of my own healing. It is happening in my life; it can happen in yours. Time and time again I have been shown that if I kept the faith, held tight to my inner prayers and continued on my healing path, miracles would take place. This I know for sure. Healing Thyself is a self-actualized miracle; it is following the pathway to the Master Plan of Optimal Wellness and the joys of life that come with it. If you are holding *Man Heal Thyself: Journey to Optimal Wellness* in your hands, you are holding a guidebook for self-transformation. You have at your fingertips and within yourself the means to participate in your own miracles; your own healing and the opportunity to become a Supreme Man of Optimal Wellness. There is a Master Plan beyond the desperate cries of brothers, sons, fathers and grandfathers. And beyond the cries and screams of the women who love them. When you consciously choose to Heal Thyself in balance – wellness – righteousness (Principle of Maát), you consciously choose to participate in and enjoy the Master Plan.

INTRODUCTION

"The power to heal is within me, and I have the power to heal myself."
QUEEN AFUA

Man, *Heal Thyself: Journey to Optimal Wellness* takes a man on a wellness journey through the anatomy of his body and its relationship to his mind and spirit. He is encouraged to take this journey to systematically and holistically detoxify from dis-eases in order to evolve from brokenness to wholeness. We will start by examining the physical anatomy of man. We examine the heart of man's body and the heart of man's soul. We will describe how to utilize the qualities in plants, earth, water, air and fire for use as tools of restoration. We are on a mission of self-defense and self-mastery to create transformation of body mind and soul for health and longevity.

The Man Heal Thyself journey to Optimal Wellness is a twelve-week excursion to examine and recalibrate your inner and outer wellness from the bottom of your feet to the top of your head. On these pages are exercises to detoxify from the lifestyle habits that contribute to numb hands and cracked toes, premature balding, jaundiced eyes, arthritic bones, high blood pressure, swollen legs, labored asthmatic breathing, impacted colon, prolapsed bladder, conditions related to diabetes, impotent prostate, failed kidneys and low back pain, back and more dis-eases. *Man Heal Thyself* addresses the broken-down spirits and war scars, such as, lack of vision attitudes, emotional constipation, unresolved parental resentment and failed relationships. These spiritual and emotional conditions are symptoms of the toxicity trapped in the physical cells; they keep you from realizing to your higher self.

I offer *Man Heal Thyself* as a healing balm to take you in and make you over. *Man Heal Thyself* contains suggestions for naturally eliminating the burdens of dis-ease from man's mind, body and soul; leaving him intact, loved-up and reborn. The text herein teaches man how to holistically recognize the natural connection between his hip bone and his knee bone; his crown and his feet. He will learn how to restore wellness to and from his mind, his heart, his body and his spirit. As a Holistic Body Temple Architect he will learn to strategically build himself from a wounded man of dis-ease to a vibrant Heal Thyself Man of Wellness, to a dynamic, and radiant Supreme Man of with high-frequency and optimal wellness. Following the strategies proposed in *Man, Heal Thyself: Journey to Optimal Wellness* will create the transformation of himself. In just twelve weeks, one season, a man will journey on a path of Emerald Green Natural Living and end the pattern of dis-ease. A man healing himself will learn to break free from a toxic, destructive, lifestyle that up to now has been unbreakable cycles frequently plaguing his family's bloodline from generation to generation. This book provides exercises for developing new habits to help you to eliminate age-old blockages (dis-eases) to your physical, mental, emotional, psychological, and social wellness. Upon reading *Man Heal Thyself* you can look forward to traveling on a new pathway towards the resurrection of your wellness.

A wounded man who wants to grow into Heal Thyself Man must first know: that man is not by nature a bastard, a liar, a thief, a con-man, an abuser, a male whore who is armed and dangerous. He is not naturally an out-of-control species who lacks discipline and divinity. To grow into a Heal Thyself Man, one must discover the true nature of a Heal Thyself Man is one of power, beauty, harmony and radiance. A Heal Thyself Man is one who is mentally, physically, emotionally, socially, and sexually balanced. A Heal Thyself Man is in harmony with himself, and with the Divine in himself. He is in harmony with nature and therefore, in harmony with all his relationships. The essence and origin of such a Man was born out of the Original Man from the First Civilization, and his name is Nefer Atum, The Lotus Man. The Lotus Man is the pure one (clean) the beautiful one (radiant), the illuminated one (intelligent), and the mighty one (powerful). Like the lotus, a man makes the same evolution; he journeys out of the "mud" of the challenges and the lessons. Through the purification process, through the twelve states of man he will elevate to become The Lotus Man. Like a small acorn becomes a mighty oak tree, the Man Heal Thyself principles will grow a man holistically in order to magnify his wellness and vitality. In one season, man will learn to use food and positive affirmations in the manner surgeons use scalpels and medicine. Man will restore himself to balance using the tools of nature.

During one season, twelve weeks, a man will travel through twelve the stages of man as he performs self-healing detoxification and rejuvenation exercises. During each stage he will focus on a specific checkpoint of his physical and meta-physical being. In this text I cite these checkpoints as the Aritu. Within the first seven weeks, by using Arti 1-7, he will overcome some of the dis-eases of The Wounded Man. He will be able to release the yoke of excessive weight and the burden of high blood pressure that comes with it. He can begin to regain his sexual potency and restore his memory. In the Man Heal Thyself stages of his development he will begin focusing on and creating healthier relationships. By activating the wellness exercises of the next five Aritu (Arit 8 – 12), man will rise from Man Heal Thyself to a Supreme Man of Optimal Wellness - the highest frequency of wellness.

Throughout the twelve-week season, man will re-mold his body to health and longevity as one would mold clay. On a daily basis he will be using natural wellness tools such as, visualization exercises, freedom walks, affirmations and herbs and clay compounds. Diligently he will align himself with the four elements and begin developing new habits. He will begin eating and living a green lifestyle that supports optimal wellness. His use of zone therapy will include eliminating the meta-physics of dis-ease and reaching for the meta-physics of Wellness in his life. In twelve weeks, with the support of the Heal Thyself Wellness formulas and techniques, man will strategically rise beyond dietary enemies and toxic social medications (i.e. drugs, alcohol, and cigarettes) as he raises his body, mind, and spiritual frequencies. To embark on a Man Heal Thyself regiment is to embark on a lifestyle to wellness. The strategies for the twelve weeks will open the gates and provide holistic instructions as the Wounded Man travels on his pathway to wellness.

WELCOME TO THE JOURNEY.

CHAPTER 1

THE WOUNDED
MAN

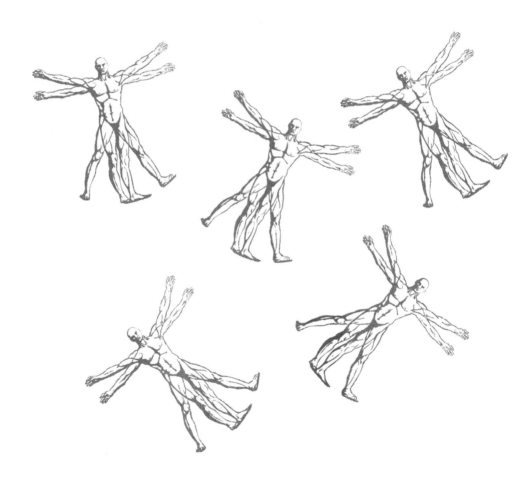

THE MILLION MAN MARCH:
THRESHOLD TO MAN HEAL THYSELF

At 7:05 on an August morning in 1995 I got a call from Bob Law –then, a WWRL Radio executive and the talk show host of "Night Talk". He said, "Congratulations, Queen, you have chosen to coordinate the fasting protocol for the Million Man March. On October 16th, this year, one million men are going to march into Washington, DC to gather on the steps of the capital of the United States of America."

Minister Louis Farrakhan had proposed the idea of a day of atonement to what became the national organization committee for the Million Man March. As a member of the national committee, Bob Law organized and became chair of the organizing committee in New York State. He introduced New York State community and religious leaders, who included Reverend Johnny Ray Youngblood, Reverend Calvin Butts and many other visionaries, to Minister Farrakhan. Minister Farrakhan charged them to encourage their male constituents to become part of the march. Meanwhile, at the meeting, my good friend Dianna Pharr suggested, "The men going to the Million Man March could stronger if they fasted before the event. She reminded the committee, "Queen Afua specializes in fasting and liberation through purification." Together, Bob Law and Dianna Pharr proposed that a fasting component become part of the Million Man March agenda. Minister Farrakhan gave his verbal support to the suggestion to have the men fast; other committee members agreed. Bob Law was calling me to tell me to prepare a fasting proposal for the Million Man March. I realized that as they raised their voices as one in unity, redemption and atonement, it would resound around the world. None of them would ever be the same! I was breathless.

I accepted at that very moment. This was the answer to a twenty-six year old prayer. Bob Law knew I had healed myself, holistically. He knew that I was a certified Holistic Health Consultant and had created a 21-Day Fasting Program. He, himself had been the one to push me to write Heal *Thyself for Health and Longevity*. He knew I believed that if my people could be exposed to holistic fasting and detoxification on a mass level, we could break the chains of health disparity nationally and globally. The call that August morning in 1995 was a turning point for me. I could raise collective consciousness and we could begin to heal ourselves. Bob Law was confident in my ability to prepare the proposal for a million men to fast. The supreme honor to write the fasting proposal had me rise before dawn for four days to channel from on High and to prepare. My prayers were to create a program that not only would affect the million men, but eventually would have an impact on the state of all men's wellness. Here was the chance to make a massive change and the world would watch as we healed ourselves and became loving examples of the power in nature to Heal Thyself.

I designed a fasting program for three lifestyle levels so that each man could have access atonement according to his awareness and experience with holistic fasting and detoxification. As they say, *water would seek its own level.*

Fasting Level 1 – fast from negativity. The man and his family in support would fast and detox one month before the day of the Million Man March. Men on Level 1 would fast from viewing negative television (programs focusing on violence) in order to focus on restoring the brain and mind to wholeness. They would not curse or use foul language among themselves and their friends, nor with their family. They would avoid using drugs, alcohol and cigarettes for a month. They would also refrain from eating beef and pork.

Fasting Level 2 – The man and his family in support would follow the Level 1 Fast. Additionally, they would fast from "fast food", junk food, processed food and all meat including chicken and fish.

Fasting Level 3 – The man and his family in support would follow the steps in the Level 1 Fast and Level 2 Fast. Additionally, according to the health challenges of the fasters they would perform a therapeutic total liquid fast using specific freshly pressed green juices to rejuvenate and specific freshly squeezed fruit juices to detoxify. Level 3 fasters would drink eight be 8 glasses of water a day to assist with colon detoxification. They would perform hydrotherapy home baths and drink herbal compounds accordingly to their wellness needs.

I prepared a document and presented it to the New York City Million Man March organization board. All board members agreed except one. The objector strongly recommended that a fast of this magnitude would be best if prepared by a committee of medical doctors as opposed to a holistic practitioner. Bob Law said I was the best one for the job and fought for my proposal to be accepted. The objector won the battle against my proposal and although they paid attention some of my suggestions, the men lost the holistic fasting program I had prepared. It was a sad time for wellness, nevertheless, a powerful time for unity of the men. On October 16, 1995 I sent my two sons to Washington, DC, for I knew the Million Man March would empower them for life.

Word got back to me about my sons from my brother who had accompanied his nephews to Washington, DC. Although they had not been given an official platform, Supa Nova Slom, my eldest son, with his brother Ali by his side had stood up for wellness that day. They had not been included on the agenda of speakers, however they shouted out to the men at the march, "Don't eat from the fast food restaurants and food stands... Men, we are here to atone and detox, not to poison ourselves...Million Men, let this be a day of healing, not harming ourselves... We are what we eat." Supa Nova gathered a group of young men to go into the fast food spots (I call fast food restaurants *corporate kitchens* – See my book *The City of Wellness*) to encourage the men at the march not to eat *death.* (Around our kitchen table I had trained my sons to fight for wellness; to fight for life. So, from very young ages they were aware of the health disparity of the Black Man and the relationship of that disparity eating food that was not life-giving.)That day, during the Million Men March, Supa Nova, at age 18 and his brother, Ali, at age 13 stood up for wellness. They were present and advocating for wellness with their voices raised high: "Man Heal Thyself, Man Heal Thyself!"

Through the efforts of my sons and Bob Law and his wife, Muntu Law and other believers in wellness, nearly twenty years after the seeds were planted deeply in the ground, the Man Heal Thyself vision is coming to pass. The time is to "Purify or Die." Prophecy says this is the time of the end of the world.

I say, it is the time for new beginnings.

THE WOUNDED MAN

The reason a man would seek to heal himself is because in some many ways he has been wounded. This chapter takes a look at five types of men who are wounded in their physical, mental, spiritual and social states of being. These wounds include the decline of man, the blockages in man, the issue of being "half a man", the attitudes of a man who lacks in many parts of his life. Men can overcome these states of dis-ease. Once a man is honest with his emotions, then and only then can he transform himself to a natural, brilliant, loving, powerfully balanced man-state. He will be able to restore and secure his breath of life. Through the 12-week journey he will learn how to restore and rejuvenate wellness to the twelve Aritu (checkpoints) so that eventually he can achieve optimal wellness socially, emotionally and spiritually.

THE COMMON MAN

"Don't be common." Our mother would say this to my brothers and I whenever, we, as children, "acted up". According to my mother, being "common" was the worst thing my brothers and I could ever be. But, The Common Man doesn't have to be "acting up"; generally, he is a man who is normal and average. His life is complacent and uneventful; he lives safely in the bosom of mediocrity. A Common Man has Lack Syndrome that keeps his life deficient, uneventful and unfulfilled. A Common Man is a Wounded Man because his limited vision and low energy cause him to suffer from physical, emotional, social, sexual, and financial challenges. He is trapped in toxic, low frequency, stressful, out of control, relationships. A Common Man is disconnected from his inner and outer power; mentally, physically and spiritually. You must be willing to overcome The Common Man is who in order to reach Man Heal Thyself of Health and Longevity to the Supreme Man of Optimal Wellness.

THE NEGATIVE ALPHA MAN

The phone rings, a man has called 718 221 HEAL. He says, *"Queen I heard your presentation in Atlanta, GA at The Shrine of The Black Madonna. You spoke about The Negative Alpha Man. I felt you were talking about and to me. In a quivering voice, the man on the phone said, "I don't want to be that man anymore. I keep losing my mates because of The Negative Alpha Man influence and I want to change. I have a mate at present and I hope The Negative Alpha Man didn't already run her away like the others. It's like I can't control myself, like another me takes over. I start off as a positive Alpha Man and then the moment I feel secure in the relationship The Negative Alpha Man kicks in and I begin dominating and controlling the relationship. Queen, please help me, I want to be healed."*

By the time I finished speaking with him he was ready to claim his true self and take on the Wellness Warrior that would walk him through the 12 States of manhood.

An Alpha Man in a negative state, is a dominating, aggressive, pushy, short-fused, controlling, manipulating, 'Know it All'. He is verbally oppressive and abusive and maybe even physically violent. The Negative Alpha Man believes it's "his way or the highway." He's egotistically driven. The Negative Alpha Man does not share his full heart for fear of hurt and he suppresses his problems and pain. The suppressed pain lashes out and in a backhand slap to the woman, who, according to him, "talks too much." He hides himself in silence in hopes that no one finds out about his rage.

The Negative Alpha Man keeps his woman "in check" and under control, and keeps her family and friends at a distance. The Negative Alpha Man views his mate as his property and wants to ensure that she is not influenced by what he views as 'outside forces'. The Negative Alpha Man has the skill to present himself as a Positive Alpha Man to the public but behind the door dwells The Negative Alpha Man. His wife is afraid, his children are distant and his friends are concerned.

The Negative Alpha Man is emotionally unavailable to his wife after the honeymoon wears off. He pats his children on their heads, disciplines them, contributes to their upkeep; but don't expect him to rock, hold, or cradle them. After all he provided the seed of them—that's enough, according to The Negative Alpha Man

The Negative Alpha Man and the Positive Alpha Man do have one thing in common. Both believe that crying to release pain, hurt and disappointment, is a sign of weakness. If a Man is able to cry when needed, he will be able to purify his heart. With the flow of his tears, his water element will become un-dammed. This will cause his high blood pressure to lower and prevent heart attacks and depression.

The Negative Alpha Man commonly works himself to death. Heart attacks and strokes are natural occurrences in The Negative Alpha Man. When a man treats his wife as his child and his children as his possessions, he is at the height of being the negative Alpha Man.

If, as a chronic Negative Alpha Man, you meet your reflection—a Negative Alpha Woman and you want to save yourself, don't walk, RUN for your life onto the journey to Man Heal Thyself.

THE ANGRY OLD MAN

The Angry Old Man has a special chair that he sits in night after night. The chair has a dent in it because he's been sitting in it for so long. He watches television where other people win the game of life, or lose the girl, or fight for their beliefs while he sits his life away. He lost control and he can't seem to get out of the funk. He is stuck in the complacency that surrounds him. The Angry Old Man is a tired and depressed man that could be as young as a teenager of 18 or as old as 88 years of age. An Angry Old Man is an attitude. The Angry Old Man is about a man who has not fulfilled his life and whose dreams have been deferred. His hopes have not been realized and his visions have yet to be manifested. As a result The Angry Old Man feels empty of self-satisfaction and full of anger and regrets. He is angry because he has not been heard, he feels unappreciated, and is not recognized for his gifts and talents. He is angry and old because his heart is filled with rage, hate, disgust, dismay, resentment and hurt resulting from unhealed wounds of the past. He is angry and old because unbeknownst to himself, he has created a box that he lives in with a sign on it that reads, "Stay Away! Love doesn't live here!" People around him get it and they stay clear of The Angry Old Man. This only makes him angrier for it's the aloneness that causes the anger to fester, causing The Angry Old Man to harbor tension that even keeps The Angry Old Man away from himself—lacking self-love.

The Angry Old Man's state was planted in the sperm and in the ovum at the conception long before he was born and was passed down over generations. The Angry Old Man's state continued to grow when, as a small boy and as a youth, Daddy didn't hug him or Mother ignored him, or both parents worked so hard that they didn't have much "lap-time" to give to him. Maybe he wasn't held as a baby at his mother's breast or in his father's arms and therefore he suffers starvation for healthy-touch. Perhaps he was a latch-key kid, or lived in a single-parent home where he waited for Daddy who never returned home. He might have experienced many false promises from the elders that were in fact broken, so as a youth his heart shut down to protect him from more pain. He may have even been sexually assaulted, and so, as he carried his lack of love into his adulthood the assault absolutely had to be a secret. The Angry Old Man runs away—from his children, his wife, his friends; himself. He seldom has anything good to speak on because he's so filled with what he feels—hurt turned into anger. The Angry Old Man could show up as demonic, for indeed, what has happened is that the anger has turned in on itself and "possessed" the host.

The Angry Old Man has a special chair (or couch) in his house that becomes his Throne of Anger. As a 'couch potato' The Angry Old Man sits and absorbs reflections of the pain in his own life while he stares at the lives of others—in pain—on the 5 and 6 and all day and all night o'clock news. He adds the bad news, sad news, violent news to his own pain and so The Angry Old Man's inner condition gets worse. The Angry Old Man ages quickly, his heart is weakened, broken and heavy and he is therefore a candidate for a sudden heart attack or slow-to-come stroke. For The Angry Old Man, The Common Man and The Negative Alpha Man there is a way out by bravely taking the journey through the twelve states of Man Heal Thyself to A Supreme Man of Optimal Living.

THE SEXUALLY ADDICTIVE MAN

The sexual addictive man is obsessed by a dark spirit that "rides" his mind, heart and body. This spirit can possess the rest and the best of men. I witnessed that some really powerful men who, as religious leaders, social justice leaders, cultural leaders, martial arts masters, presidents, CEOs and artistic leaders have succumbed to the sexual addictive spirit. On the news we read and hear about these addictions as headline stories. I've witnessed men of nobility, act as hustlers, pimps, sex fiends and addicts with total disregard for their partner's body and/or emotions.

As The Sexually Addictive Man, an educated, intelligent and otherwise "do-good" man gets so caught up that, even though he is more likely than not to get caught 'out there with his pants down', he will give in to his addiction with sex. And he will do so, anywhere—in a lavish four star hotel or a run down, at-the-end-of-town motel; in a truck or a tractor trailer at a highway rest stop, in the oval office, in a back alley, in his car, in the red light district. Some men have sex night and day in cyber space, empowered by a heavy diet of girly or manly magazines and DVDS. Even though he might get caught by his wife, his lover, his community or his nation, The Sexually Addictive Man will take his chances because he is an addict. He can't say, "No." He can't stop, he's out of control. He's got to get what he wants, when he wants it; he just has to have it regardless of the circumstances and consequences. These men will risk losing their children or damaging their reputation. Some sexually addicted men are sex offenders who hunt women or other men or children. Regardless of the circumstances they will seek out their prey in order to satisfy their addiction. Some addicts need to have flesh to flesh touch, so badly, that they are willing to have sex without protection which makes them automatically willing to spread viruses they may have. Like playing Russian roulette with a loaded pistol to the head, they take their chances with their partner's life. With their irresponsible behavior, these perpetrators not only leave behind Womb-war casualties (angry women), but also, they acquire insurmountable karmic debt for which payment will be called, usually in the most unfortunate turn of events. Remember, for every action there is equal reaction. Some addicts have rotating girlfriends always keeping a warm vagina on standby. Some addicts set up a polygamy stable under the guise of cultural and religious righteousness. They have a different woman in bed with them Monday through Sunday. The women not only performs sexual duties for him, but also cooks, washes the dishes, cleans, does laundry and performs child care duties.

Some Sexually Addictive Men ejaculate so often that their sperm is weak and malnourished. This results in a debilitated brain, weak cells, and a challenged immune system. As The Sexually Addictive Man continues his destructive behavior to others he may suffer from impotency at an earlier age than expected. In addition, if the addicts are consumers of fried foods, junk food and drugs, they become carriers of toxic sperm that poisons their partner and produces dilapidated offspring.

Whether you were bottle-fed rather than breastfeed or your father or your mother was not in the home or you were sexually abused as a child and beat up emotionally by women, men, lovers, partners, and mates, you can overcome the dis-ease of using your penis as an extension of your pain and a lethal weapon, Yes, you can heal. Man, take the walk of Man Heal Thyself and be whole, stop passing your tension, your pollution, and your past misgivings onto your partner and calling it "sex" or "love" as you work out your inner dis-harmony inside your partner's body.

Man, save your life; elevate; raise your frequency; purge the hurt and dis-ease from your body and your mind and your spirit. Be still, as you restore peace and balance and control into your life. With each day of self-transformation, bear witness to a life of love, rather than lust; peace, rather than war.

THE BROKEN MAN

Monday, at noon. Lady Prema, my dear friend, called me and said, "I am working with a brother here who is in urgent need of healing." I said, "Give him herbs and a clay pack; have him lie down on the floor on his back and put his legs up at a 45° angle against the wall. Give him green drinks until he feels like he's saturated in green drinks." I knew my friend knew how to do what I was telling her to do. "He'll come around in 24 hours," I said. And this, he did.

To you, Lady Prema's friend, and all your brothers, I dedicate *Man Heal Thyself!* The power to heal is within you.

A strong man came to me for consultation. His grandfather had just passed away. His grandfather had nurtured him throughout his life; they were close. His grandfather had been the root and the rock of the family. Upon his grandfather's transition into the spirit world, this young man's bottom fell out. The women in his family broke down all around him, weeping and wailing. He was the only man left in his family. He was frightened of the responsibility of being in this position. As a rule, men do not outlive women; and this is unfortunately and certainly the norm in African American community. In the average Black family the men die between 45 – 65 years of age. The women live until between onto 75 – 85 years of age. Meanwhile, the women live through hysterectomies, mastectomies, cancer, depression and loneliness we live through it all without men.

Why is this?

Below are some of the conditions contributing to the early death of Black men in the United States. Statistics will vary, but these conditions contributing to the early death also can be applied to men of African descent throughout the African Diaspora. Within *Man Heal Thyself* you will read of the health disparity status suffered by African American men. All too frequently, in large numbers, Black men are suffering from heart attacks, stroke, prostate cancer and high blood pressure. Within *Man Heal Thyself* are holistic preventions to these and other wellness challenges. Men, Heal Thyself over 21 days and receive 40 – 50% better wellness. Follow the path to Supreme Men of Optimal Wellness.

- 17.5% of the unemployed are Black men
- 44% of the population in shelters are homeless Black men
- 37% of Black men are obese
- 72% of Black men come from single parent homes
- 36% of Black men are alcoholic
- 45% of Black men are in prison
- 31% of gang activity exists in the urban community of the Black family
- Unknown – the percentage of the Black men who were sexually abused in their youth. The misplaced shame they harbor prevents usually them from sharing this tragic information. Therefore, the numbers are difficult to calculate and the healing process is delayed or often never even begins.
(Statistical data obtained from several sources. See Reference Section.)

I challenge The Broken Man to take the Journey to recapture, restore, re-awaken yourself to wholeness. Give yourself daily wellness care, so that you may live long and strong with your families. Overcome The Broken Man and become a Supreme Man of Optimal Wellness and enjoy longevity as your reward.

CHAPTER 2

ENTER THE WELLNESS WARRIORS

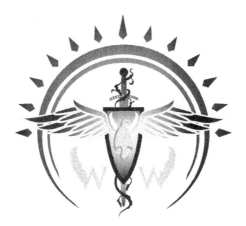

THE WELLNESS WARRIOR SHIELD

The Wellness Warrior Protective Shield contains:
The feather of Maát
represents balance, truth and justice.
The sword of Bes
represents cutting away corruptible matter
to move beyond limitations.
The Falcon, king of the air
soars above adversity
represents leadership and self mastery.
The vegetation within
represents rejuvenation.
The surrounding circle
represents a continuum of inner and outer power.
Rays around the shield
represent radiant light.

THE WELLNESS WARRIOR MAN

The Wellness Warrior creed is simply, "Purify or Die."
SUPA NOVA SLOM

We recognize and salute The Wellness Warrior Man and Healing Champion Man who have traveled beyond the state of The Common Man. You are the men on the Man Heal Thyself journey. You are still on the Quest to becoming Supreme Men of Optimal Wellness.

The Wellness Warrior Man is diligently on his path to wellness. It takes your full force, your full attention and your convictions to break the cycle of toxic mental, physical, sexual, and dietary addictions and tap into your inner wholeness. The Wellness Warrior Man has come to the awareness that in order to Heal Thyself, he must fight to receive and maintain his wellness. The Wellness Warrior fights to overcome a toxic lifestyle.

In order to maintain a healthy and vibrant life style, The Wellness Warrior lives detoxification and rejuvenation techniques, daily. He protects himself from falling prey to toxic living with drugs, alcohol and tobacco, as well as flesh food, junk food and micro-waved food. The Wellness Warrior transforms himself, by any means necessary, to become enlightened and whole in body, mind, and spirit. The Wellness Warrior is a force to be reckoned with; he will fight for his wellness. His battle tools are determination, commitment and conviction. The Wellness Warrior not only will defend his right to live a healthy vibrant life, but he also fights for the wellness restoration and rejuvenation of his family, friends, associates, and community. He a warrior for the global population's right to wellness.

Just as Bes (The Spiritual Guardian of Evolution and Transformation), takes the sword and cuts away corruptible matter and disease, The Wellness Warrior uses his spiritual sword to cut away issues and desires that diminish his life force. He will place the feather of Maát (balance and harmony) over the wounds as he transforms into the hawk and flies above all adversity to his Optimal Wellness.

I say to The Wellness Warrior Man with the conviction to be made whole, "Pick up your shield and sword as you cut away obstructions and continue your journey to defend wellness for your self and others."

MY SONS, WELLNESS WARRIORS

I am a mother who exposed my sons, Supa Nova Slom and Ali to many disciplines to strengthen them as they grew from boys to teens to adult men. As a Wellness Warrior Mother, I ran a Wellness Warrior Boot Camp. My sons attended cultural-alternative, vegetarian schools. They studied various forms of martial arts including, Jujitsu, Karate, Tai Chi, Shalom Temple Martial Arts and body building. Culturally conscious men were their teachers. They were taught Yoruba spiritually from their blood father, David Torain and alchemy from their first stepfather, Rev. Valentine. They learned Khamitic Living Legacy from Sen Ur Ankh Ra Semahj Se Ptah, their second stepfather. My first born took his training to the streets on a mission to unify The Crips and The Bloods in the hood. He went to teach them ways of the wellness warrior spirit; to show them to how to live, rather than to die.

Supa Nova fearlessly walked into the hood with the feather of Maát in his hair and the ankh symbol for life in his hand. He carried a red rag symbolizing The Bloods and a blue rag symbolizing The Crips. My son's friend from childhood jumped onto the train tracks and took his life after fighting with his girlfriend. Our neighborhood friend had one brother who was locked away in prison for fifteen and another brother who is presently serving life in prison. A third friend has returned to prison repeatedly during his young life. For thirty-five years of his life Supa Nova's served at our family wellness center; Ali likewise has been serving for thirty years. Their entire lives were dedicated to living vegetarian, vegan and chlorophyllian lifestyles, which served as examples in communities at home and abroad. Supa Nova Slom is in the Army now. I've trained him and his brother the art of discipline all their lives. Ali serves in the army of wellness known as the Queen Afua Wellness Institute.

My sons and I were talking at the kitchen table. They honored me by knighting me The Wellness Warrior Mother. They recognized that I had been there to protect and defend them. I was thinking how my efforts had helped to prepare them to stand up and Man Heal Thyself principles at the Million Man March and throughout the events of their lives so far. I am blessed to have raised Wellness Warrior Men.

THE HEALING JUGGERNAUTS

We recognize and salute The Healing Juggernaut Man. You have been on the front line of wellness. You have been devoted to 'the work' for over ten years; some of you for over thirty and even forty years. Be of courage; be inspired. All that you have contributed to raising the people has not gone in vain. Your healing hands have surrounded the world.

The Healing Juggernauts carried the natural medicine within them, as if it were in their loins and shared their path of wellness with the multitude. First, they transformed themselves and then they reached out to assist all others who were on a quest to take back their lives. The time has come, 2012 and beyond, where the masses are beginning to awaken and witness the wellness shift. The Business man, the Cultural man, the Spiritualist, the Health Activist man, have come for products and to workshops, seminars and consultations, seeking wellness solutions. Now, the Hustler Man and the brother from 'Around the Way' Man are coming for wellness. They are 'busting down the door'. They want to get off the drugs, cigarettes and alcohol that are poisoning their blood and stifling their thinking. They are seeking to stop the consumption of dead and infested flesh that's causing cancer and a short life expectancy. The Wellness Warrior Healing Juggernauts are pulling them onto the path of wellness.

The men have been crying out in silence for help to be saved, to be whole and to overcome the life of toxicity, which is no life at all. The men who lack of how to achieve wellness are coming to The Healing Juggernauts. They are seeking help to release themselves from the addictions that has chained them to their demise. The Juggernaut Man will help men come out of the dark alley. The Juggernaut Man will rescue the men who use over-the-counter drugs for temporary relief from toxic symptoms and, who, when the effects of the drugs wear off need more potent substances to numb the pain. Often these substances have been more over-the-counter drugs, illegal drugs, toxic food and toxic sexual encounters. Still, the hurt didn't go away. The men have had enough and are ready to 'take the monkey off their back. '

The Holistic Medicine Men from the four directions, North, South, East and, West, walk in the footprints of the eldest ancestors to help the man in the midst of body, mind, spiritual, and relationship disparity. The Healing Juggernaut Men, have stayed the course, held their ground and paid their dues in order to be master healers. Be encouraged, Healing Juggernaut Man. We know for many it has been difficult to keep the faith. Remove your ego and continue to help the men who are bleeding now, and have been for generations. Help them to break the chains that have destroyed lives in the form of poor dietary habits. Dis-eases of body, mind and spirit have plagued generations from the days of plantation slavery to these new days of prison industrial slavery. Healing Juggernaut Man we call upon you to help free the parents who conceive and birth sick babies. We look forward to the birth of well babies, who as returning giants can save humanity. The people have faith in The Healing Juggernaut Man.

Master Healers, Brothers, Fathers, Elders, Men in Wellness, you fought the system and you won. You stood for truth in the line of fire and did not bend. You held on tight for the people so that they could recover. You, the Healing Juggernaut have walked the pathway and have become the living legacy of great, mighty, wise men. I feel profound gratitude for the spiritual architects, Wellness bricklayers and holistic pyramid builders. You diligently worked the forces of nature as you packed, wrapped, smudged, sweated and fed natural foods and herbs to the men and families in need. Through the laying on of hands and your prayers you helped the seekers of Wellness. From the United States to the Caribbean, from the United Kingdom to Africa and Brazil, to those I met face to face, and those I met in spirit, I thank you. Healing Juggernauts who carry knowledge and do the work, we appreciate you.

THANK YOU, DOCTOR DAVIDSON

Doctor Ronald Davidson, a friend and colleague, a medical doctor, and a holistic physician passed on, into the Ancestral realm in the winter of 1997; he was 54 years, young. The entire community admired his laser sharp mind and his hard work, as well as the bond he had to his patients. In his Brooklyn and Manhattan clinics he had merged allopathic with holistic practices decades before it became fashionable to do so. Doctor Davidson was a The Healing Juggernaut Man.

It was Dr. Davidson who opened his doors to me to work in his clinic 25 years ago, when I was but a neophyte in the Holistic Health field. Forgetting his own needs, he quickly and quietly moved from patient to patient, to give them all he had in him from the best of his allopathic and holistic knowledge. Year in and year out, he took care of us. After writing a prescription for diabetic patients he would insist they begin the exercise portion of their healing right then and there on the stationery bicycle in his clinic. He understood the importance of cultural celebration through music and dance and artistic expression and set up "concerts" performed and attended by his patients. The concerts were healing forthem and the community at large. Dr. Davidson fully absorbed the role of teaching the community to Heal Thyself. The fact that he never said, "No," to any of us caused him to live his life as a Healing Juggernaut. His decision to help us find the "yes" to our wellness may have cost him his life and cost his family and the community the loss of a dear and profound man of medicine.

To The Healing Juggernaut Man, to the all the men on your path to wellness, do not let the life and work of Dr. Davidson be in vain. In his honor and memory, pick up your shield and be encouraged to be a Heal Thyself Man valiantly on your journey to Optimal Wellness.

Rest in peace Dr. Davidson; I dedicate to you, the day to day lifestyle of Man Heal Thyself.

EMERALD GREEN HOLISTIC PRACTITIONERS

Emerald Green Holistic Practitioners have studied and are certified in the principles and practices of a holistic lifestyle. Emerald Green Holistic Practitioners are Wellness Warriors because they are ready to defend the wellness of their clients/students.

SAVED MY LIFE

Peace and blessings to all of my wellness warrior brothers. My name is De'Arcy BA-RA and Man Heal Thyself has changed my life. I come from a family of very strong Queens. My grandmother and mother raised me, so I know the power of a woman and the healing that takes place when there is no resistance.

I once ate pork, beef, junk food, fast food, micro-waved food, EVERY DAY! My mother had to work two jobs so I had to survive the best way I knew how. I read Queen Afua's *Heal Thyself*, and it changed my life. After witnessing my grandmother's illness, my mother's struggle, and my own sister's womb being taken right in front of me – all relating to an unhealthy lifestyle, I had to learn and quickly! As my sister screamed for a ride to the hospital every month, and my grandmother could not leave her bed, I said 'THAT'S IT! NO MORE!! I will awaken the healer within and Heal Thyself, and my Queens".

Queen Afua saved my life. I am now an Emerald Green Holistic Practitioner and a strict vegan. My family understands that liberation comes through purification. Man, Heal Thyself is my guide, my sword, my protection.

De'Arcy BA-RA
Journalist/Artist

GRATITUDE FOR HEALING

Through my study as an Emerald Green Holistic Practitioner, I've become conscious that, I am a seer – I see a lot of life much clearer. I accept that I am a healer, but before I could talk about healing, I had to start healing with the "Man in the Mirror". In order to guide others to Wellness I had to be sure that my health was intact. I had to Heal Thyself and become a temple, clean and pure. I drink and eat foods that are green and raw. With every sip and bite, I add years to my life. I am Emerald Green straight to the heart. I will not part from the Emerald Green life. I'm not a flexitarian, vegan, or vegetarian. I'm a straight up Emerald Green Chlorophyllion.

I give thanks and praise to the Most High and the ancestors. I give thanks and praise to my mother for being the vessel through which I returned. She taught me the importance of a holistic lifestyle, how to be truly spiritual and introduced the teachings of Queen Afua to my brother and sister and me. I give thanks and praise to my wife and children for travelling with me on this journey of wellness. I give thanks and praise to Queen Afua for your teachings and guidance and also bestowing upon me the title of Emerald Green Holistic Practitioner and Supa-Man. May the Most High continue to use you as a vessel for healing. We've only just begun. Now the real work comes, because we are Wellness Warriors who have a mission to fulfill. Queen Afua, you are the Queen of Green.

Hotep,
Brother Heru Jamal
Security Harlem Hospital

I WILL NOT DIE

I will not die while I am living, numbing myself, burying the pain.

I will fully live a life of healing.

I will not die. I will live, while living.

I will not die from violence or a tragic accident.

I will not die because I didn't eat right.

I will not die from living a toxic life.

I will not die from any unhealthy reason.

I will not die from not fasting every new season.

I will not die because my body is purified and my healthy glow shows it.

I will not die because my body is the temple that holds my spirit.

I will not die because I'm one with the most high and I know it.

I will not die because my spirit is immortal.

I will not die because my soul travels back and forth through the heavenly portals.

I will not die because I've learned my life lessons.

I will live in the spiritual,

So when the time comes that I transcend my physical,

I will not die.

These are simple truths that I can't deny.

These are the reasons

I will not die.

By Heru Jamal

Queen's Response to *I Will Not Die*

As man grows in age the parts of the body will breakdown if they have not been protected by a wellness lifestyle. Disease mounts, as one, body systems shut down and body parts are cut away while the man is still alive. Men who smoke, drink, snort and shoot-up drugs, and who consume toxic foods and constantly have non-love-giving sexual experiences are inviting death sooner than later.

The early signs of death are arthritis, diabetes, prostate cancer, Alzheimer's, depression and low libido. A toxic lifestyle eats away at the body, mind, and soul.

Man, Heal Thyself and live fully. Walk strong in spirit and enjoy loving yourself. Learn your lessons and forgive your past. Thank your parents for carrying you to full term. DO NOT die while living. Instead, bond with your brothers in Wellness. Open your heart, offer gratitude out loud, form circles of healing. Spread the love. But most importantly, DO NOT die while living. Affirm daily, "I Will Not Die. I Will Live."

Queen Afua

WITNESSES TO WELLNESS

The Witnesses to Wellness have studied Man Heal Thyself and applied the principles to their own lives. In other words, they studied and applied and are qualified to testify. Some speak here.

I JUST WANNA TESTIFY

When I first met the Queen I knew she would take a part in changing my life. One reason was because she spoke life and promoted life. SO MANY of us want to live long, yet we intake the souls of dead animals when we eat their flesh. So many are so quick to say, "I can't give up my pork, beef, and chicken." But they don't realize that eating those things is what cuts our lives short. Queen Afua's third book, *The City of Wellness: Restoring Your Health Through the Seven Kitchens of Consciousness* is where I was introduced to the deadly impact of the "Corporate kitchen" and what to do to recover from the dis-eases one can get by eating in a bad way. Queen made me aware that I could heal myself.

I salute the Queen because she was the first to talk to me about life with the solution being life. N.O.R.E follows Queen, SO SHOULD YOU!

Noreaga
Hip Hop artist

FROM DEATH TO REJUVENATION

My mother passed when I was 8 years old. As a result, I suffered great losses throughout my life. I've worked on my recovery in different programs. I didn't understand how my body worked until I found this program, Man Heal Thyself. First, I am grateful to have the blessing of successfully completing attendance for natural healing in the Man Heal Thyself Program. Queen

Afua helped me to restore my life. I didn't understand the scroll and the teachings as a daily practice until she taught me. This is why I found the Man Heal Thyself 28 Day Detoxification Program so beneficial. With Queen Afua's weekly guidance, her creation of the Man Heal Thyself Scrolls, The City of Wellness Nutrition Kitchen Laboratory Chart, and the Liberation Diet Pyramids of Wellness, I was given the tools to learn to change my eating habits. I used Queen Afua's formulas to achieve healing of my acute diabetes. At my age, 73, I'm much more alive than I was before. There is a spiritual touching that I needed, and it occurs when Queen Afua speaks. I didn't know how to change my life or my eating habits. I had no help. I knew I was detoxified after two weeks of taking Queen Afua's formulas and living the Man, Heal Thyself, natural lifestyle. All foul eliminations ceased, there was no more constipation, body odor, bad back or bad eyesight. It was ALL GONE! I am now seeing the road and reading signs while driving at night. I am also beginning the reversal of erectile dysfunction. I now sleep six to seven hours a night without getting up to urinate every two hours as I was previously required to do. Because I have had great improvements in my mental state, I am registering to re-enter the practice of law. I recommend to all the men that you attend the next Man Heal Thyself training. Do not miss this opportunity to rejuvenate and refresh your body, spirit and mind.

I send love to you on your journey to a healthier lifestyle.

Kenneth Hagood, Esq.

THE OPENING OF THE WAY

The first day that I came under the direct personal influence of Queen Afua and her Heal Thyself: Green Road Map to Optimal Wellness Program happened in July, 2011. I had already attended Queen Afua's City of Wellness Seminars twice at the National Black Theatre in Harlem. Without any doubt, the Queen Afua's program has been the "The Opening of the Way" for my personal healing.

Economic, social, political, intellectual and spiritual oppression has ruled over my family for generations. We consumed unhealthy food and drink daily, for many years. We grew up in the inner city of New York as a part of the working poor. We did not know why or how our profound social illnesses came about. Before the teachings of the Honorable Elijah Muhammad, author of the classic book How to Eat to Live, no one ever taught us how food made our very own deep-rooted illnesses, wickedness and sickness permanent.

Queen Afua's Heal Thyself: Green Road Map to Optimal Wellness Program and the Man Heal Thyself Wellness Program has raised my health consciousness to a higher level. I started applying her recommended approach to my daily menu. I realized that I am in the process of making a lifestyle transformation which will last for the rest of my life. My wife and I have begun the process of transforming out kitchen into a Healing Kitchen Laboratory. Queen Afua has created a chart entitled The Liberation Diet Pyramids of Wellness which outline this process.

Our family is beginning to enjoy the benefits of changing our lifestyle and healing ourselves and reaching for our optimal wellness.

Hannibal Ahmed
Historian Researcher

THE POSITIVE ALPHA MAN

A positive Alpha Man is super powerful, physically and mentally. He is strong willed and determined to win in life despite his challenges. An Alpha Man is responsible and committed to whomever or whatever he believes in. The Alpha Man takes care of his family, friends, and community. His parents are proud of him. His wife adores him and his children openly love him. The Positive Alpha Man, who is in alignment with Divine Spirit, uses his blessing of unlimited creativity to ensure financial security for himself and his family. His friends respect him and his community trusts in his profound wisdom.

You can always rely on the Alpha Man to show up, to come through and to make it happen. An Alpha Man is dependable; The Alpha Man is 'The Man'. He has strong opinions. He speaks with authority, certainty and intelligence and always assumes a leadership role. The Positive Alpha Man is well read and spiritually in tune. The Alpha Man thinks outside of the box. He is resourceful and he knows that the power to manifest whatever he needs lies within. The Positive Alpha Man builds houses, bridges, families, hearts and minds. He uplifts people and restores their lives. He is the backbone and muscle of any project. No matter what obstacles arise, he finds a way to get the job done.

Be advised that the Positive Alpha Man and the Negative Alpha Man have the same strength and energy. If the Positive Alpha Man falls off from living a positive lifestyle, he could become unfocused and his ego could become compromised by challenges; he could flip-flop into the Negative Alpha Man. Therefore, Positive Alpha Man, be vigilant to practice holistic living, daily, so that you can remain positive on the path leading to Optimal Wellness.

LIFT THEM UP

In February, 2012, for the first time, I merged the teachings from *Sacred Woman: The Guide to Healing the Feminine Mind, Body and Spirit* with the teachings from the Man Heal Thyself Program. With this combined program I travelled to participate in a retreat that was being held in the town of Idyllwild, in the Mountains of Southern California.

Midway into our retreat, the sky opened and the sun's rays shined through. The men who were attending the retreat were asked to come forward -- 'front and center' --in order to receive a charge of 'rebirthing' from the women in attendance. Among them, the women were shaman, herbalists, seekers of Maát (truth), and reiki masters, sacred artists, clinical hypnotherapists, writers, wicker women, yogini and sacred spirit women. Women who were Muslims and Khamites, Yoruba and Israelites, Buddhists and

Universalists represented several of the world's religions and spiritual philoso-
phies. They united to speak words medicine for healing the men. To prepare
for the task of rebirthing the men, the women had taken herbal tonics and
fasted, done breathing work and meditated. Collectively, we gathered our
thoughts into the words we would say to the men to reshape, remake, and
reawaken their dedication to the Man Heal Thyself.

One after the other the woman chanted these words to charge, energize
and 'rebirth' the men:

*You are protectors of the womb. You are love. You create safe space.
You are teacher. It's okay to make mistakes learn from them. You are
the protectors. You truly love women and women truly love you. You
are sons of the green mother. The light of God is in your heart. All that
you need is within you. Your wounds are healed. You are our heroes.
You are co-creators. You are beautiful. We love you, we love you....
You are appreciated. We thank you. We respect you. We hear and
understand your inner cry. Be fearless and fly. You are loving fathers
and loyal sons. You are compassionate and forgiving. You are libera-
tors. You are Divine. The Spirit Guides walk with you. You use elevated
wise judgment. You have discernment at all times. You make our world
better. You conceive responsible holy sons and daughters. You are free.
You are humble yet powerful. You protect and defend. You are righteous pure and true. You are overcoming anger and hostility. You love
us and we love you. You are a giver. The ancient ones walk with you.
You cannot fail. You are genius. You are our wellness warriors.*

CHAPTER 3

THE HEALING POWER OF THE ELEMENTS

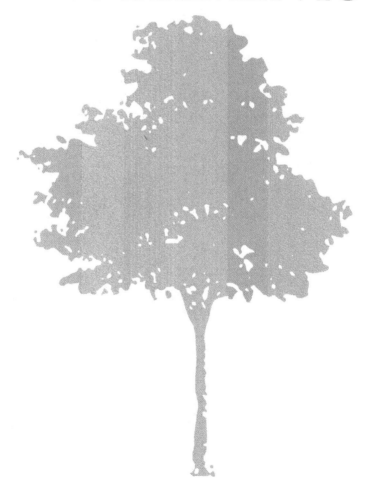

THE HEALING POWER OF THE ELEMENTS

*"We must sojourn on earth, to rediscover the light of our creation; we find that
our passage is linked to the advancement of our issues of our earthly
experience. We must discover what will bring to the highest potential
for the cooperation of the elements that compose our body, mind, and soul.
The elements of the earth sufficiently bring peace and stability
within our cellular structure. By fasting and cleansing with
The Man Heal Thyself regime we are prepared for life's journey. "*

DR PAUL BROWN BODHISE
AUTHOR OF THE URBAN SAGE:
A HOLISTIC SURVIVAL KIT
FOR THE NEW MILLENNIUM TRUTH SEEKER

THE JOURNEY
ON THE WAY TO THE
12 STATES OF MAN HEAL THYSELF

Through the anatomy of Man for 12 weeks, a season of personal commitment to wellness, man will reconstruct his body from limb to limb. Perhaps he will receive help from a wife, a friend, or a family member. Even better, maybe this Man will be able to take the time to have the time to take full responsibility for his wellness and Heal himself. He will be instructed how to use the 12 Arit energy centers (also known as chakras), the use of antiquity affirmations directly from the temple walls of the Ancient African Ancestors from the Nile Valley, herbal compounds, fasting, Heal Thyself Lifestyle practices, clay treatments, inversion exercise, zone massage, green foods, the metaphysics of wellness, journaling and the daily application of the elements: air, fire, water, and earth. Man will tap into his mighty power and so Heal Thyself. Every seven days man will activate another Arit thus building from Arit 1 – 12.

Awaken weekly, one inner conflict after the next. Each man is addressed: From Family Man, Sensual Man, Transformation Man, Lover Man, Communication Man, Intuitive Man, Universal Man, Illuminator Man, Harmonizer Man, Alchemist Man to Supreme Optimal Man, fully aware!

To explore Man Heal Thyself, we will now delve into the elements to set the tone for aligning self to wellness with the air, fire, water, and earth tools of nature. Holistic empowerment shall restore Man to grace.

THE 4 ELEMENTS OF HEALING

The Human Anatomy is a composite of elements. The elements in human body correspond with the four elements in nature: of air, fire, water and earth.

The Air element: the atomorphic – corresponds with the lungs.

The Fire element: the Sun's rays – corresponds with the bloodstream and the reproductive organs.

The Water elements: rivers, lakes, oceans – correspond to the bladder, circulatory system and the kidneys.

The Earth elements: the mountains and trees – correspond to the bones, joints, and colon.

The condition of a man's inner body is reflected in what he creates and to his relationship with himself, other people and with nature. The more vibrant and pure our inner elements are the healthier and more harmonious our lives are will be. The following information based on the elements will aid you in gaining a holistic life in body, mind, and spirit.

AIR ELEMENT

AIR ELEMENT RULES THE RESPIRATORY SYSTEM

AIR THERAPY for Optimal Wellness

Breath is life. The quality of your life is determined by the velocity of the breath. The more active the oxygen flow of the breath, the greater the mental, physical, spiritual, state of the body. We will gain healthier; relationships that are more respectful and productive.

Negative Shallow Breath:

The breath has two opposing flows. One flow is a negative direction - the breath is constrictive, shallow, and weak. The negative breath disrupts tissues, cells, bones, muscles, and nerves. Negative breathing is due primarily to stress, emotional trauma, constipation or blockages of systems throughout the body and a poor diet consisting of fast food, junk food, fried food. The negative breath creates the following dis-ease:

- Mental depression
- Shortness of breath
- Headache
- Numbness in the hands, feet, legs, etc
- Impotency
- Poor Memory
- Fatigue
- Lack of vision

How to Perform the Positive Breath:

Sit on your a comfortable chair. Align your head with your shoulders and your feet with your hips. Place your, feet flat on the floor, and your hands in your lap with palms facing upward. Align your mind with your heart, and your heart with your body.

Inhale through your nostrils as you expand your lungs and abdomen. Exhale from your nostrils as you contract your abdomen and relax your lungs.

Perform this breathing of 20 - 100 lotus fire breaths 2 - 3 times a day. If you consciously practice the full body breath, in time it will become your norm. With each breath, your body will be more and more enlivened.

Over a season increase to 1000 lotus fire breaths daily.

Perform 250 lotus fire breaths at each of these times: sunrise, midday, sunset, before bed

Movement:
Perform breathing exercises while performing Yoga, Tai Chi, Ari Ankh-KA, dance or power walking.

Formula: Breath of Life
For deeper more vibrant breaths take 2-3 drops of Heal Thyself Breath of Life formula with 8-16oz. of distilled warm water and juice of a lemon.

The result of Positive Vibrant Breathing:
The opposite of negative breathing is positive breathing. The positive breath flow is expansive, full, and strong. The positive breath brings oxygen to tissues, cells, bones, muscles, and nerves. Positive breathing will be the result of holistic eating habits, healthy relationships, and daily exercise.

FIRE ELEMENT

FIRE ELEMENT RULES THE REPRODUCTIVE SYSTEM, CIRCULATION AND THE BLOODSTREAM

FIRE THERAPY for Optimal Wellness

There is ancient Afrakan pose that is the grandmaster of all movements. The movement or pose is called "The Inversion". The Inversion Pose is to release the fire within in order to increase your circulation throughout your anatomy.

Poor Circulation:

Man stands upright most of his life. As a result, as one matures, the energy and force travel down—away from the brain—causing over time poor memory, a clogged, weak heart, low backache, prolapsed colon, bladder and prostate, and swollen knees and ankles. To perform inversion you must lie flat on your back, preferably on the floor or on a bed and place your feet against the wall at a 45 degree angle. This can be done on any flat surface where you can put against a solid surface at an incline.

How to perform inversion:

Action

Before inversion, mix equal parts of olive oil and castor oil in a bowl. Apply this blend to your legs, arms, chest, abdomen, neck, and face. While in inversion, massage this oil blend vigorously into the afore-mentioned areas concentrating on your organs—prostate, bladder, colon, and heart Do this for a full ten minutes to revitalize your body. Massage toward the heart for full revitalization effect.

- Better memory
- Strengthens heart
- Increases circulation
- Prevents prostate blockage and bladder dis-ease

Movement

Soccer, basketball, kickboxing, martial arts, roller skating. Perform 30 minutes to 1 hour daily.

The results of performing inversion:

By inverting twice a day (every sunrise and sunset) for 10 -15 minutes, man will increase blood circulation from one's crown to one's feet. Improved blood circulation which will then help to improve memory, nourish the nervous system, strengthen the heart, bladder, colon and prostate while. Performing the inversion exercise will help to prevent numbing in feet and hands.

THE INVERSION AFFIRMATION
FOR OPTIMAL CIRCULATION

You can combine the fire and breathing exercise for optimal results to the mind, body and spirit. After doing the fire breath exercise (performed at sunrise and sunset) lie flat in the bed and place your legs against the wall in a 45° angle. Relax the body and inhale and exhale as you visualize that you are recharging each part of your body with the flow of life. Recite the following Ancient Inversion Healing Affirmation from the Nile Valley Ancestors.

I am in the Utchat (Higher Consciousness, evolved mind)
Nuk am ut'at

I exist by its strength (My mind reflects my body)
Au-a em maket-s

I come forth, I shine (To go into meditation and come out vibrant)
Aq-na aux a

I have commanded my seat (I have power over my mind, my life)
Atu-ma nest-a

I maintain an exact balance (I am in harmony)
Aqa- ua

My form is inverted
Ari-a sexet

I open the door of Heaven (Balance)
Ap sba em pet

I am reborn on this day (Renewed)
Nuk nesta em hru pen

WATER ELEMENT

WATER ELEMENT RULES THE CIRCULATORY SYSTEM, BLADDER & URINARY TRACT

WATER THERAPY for Optimal Wellness

I know a man usually prefers to take showers over taking baths. Showers are quick, fast, and done. Showers wash off the funk, clean the skin, freshen the soul. Man, to heal thyself, it is strongly recommended to bathe at least 3 times per week for 20 – 30 minutes. A bath can drain the toxicity from the body and distress and anxiety from the mind. A bath rejuvenates the spirit. A bath can soften a cyst, break up plaque in the arteries, and prevent one from creating or attracting violence. Baths protect, support, and lift up the body, mind, and spirit.

I offer seven baths for you to use in order that your body can 'drink' in wellness through the millions of pores in your skin. I also offer six tonics to be taken orally for flushing toxins from the body. The bath recommendations are as follows:

BATH TONICS

Take 3 Baths Weekly

Avoid Salt & Ginger bath if you suffer from high blood pressure

1. **Dead Sea Salt or Epsom Salt – To de-stress**
    (Avoid this bath if you have high blood pressure).

    Add 1-2 lbs of bath salt to warm water. Bathe in the water. Bathe in salt bath. Drink herbal the tonic that corresponds to the target organ or situation for which you are bathing.

2. **Master Herbal Bath – To detoxify**
    Boil 4 cups of water. Turn off flame and add 4 tsp. of Master Herbal Formula to water and steep 1- 4 hours. Strain the herbs and pour the liquid into the tub. As a bath, use 3 times per week. As a tonic, drink 1 cup of Master Herbal with 12oz of H20 throughout the day until finished. It can be used daily as a tonic.

3. **Garlic Bath – To lower pressure**
    Remove 5 -10 garlic cloves from a garlic bulb. Blend with 4ozs of H20 then, pour into tub. Add 1-2 drops of Breath of Life to bath. You can drink this same solution of water garlic and Breath of Life.

4. **Lemon Bath – To break up congestion**
    Juice 5 lemons and add the juice to the bath. As a tonic, juice 1 lemon and add to 12-16 oz of H20 and drink.

5. **Ginger Bath- To improve circulation and vitality**
    Juice ½ to 1 C. of ginger from fresh ginger root then add to bath. As a tonic, take 1-2 Tbs. of fresh ginger with 12-16oz of warm H20 and drink.

6. **Organic Apple Cider Vinegar Bath – To break up congestion**
    Add ½ to 1 C. of OACV to bath. As a tonic, add 1-2 Tbs. of OACV to 12-16oz of H20 and drink.

7. **Bladder wrack, Fennel, chickweed herb- Anti swelling in legs, face, hand, ankles, kidneys, etc**

Add 1-2 tsp. of each herb to 1qt. H20, Steep overnight, strain pour into tub. Reserve some of this tonic to drink as you bathe.

How to use the Water Element to Cleanse:

Formula

Take 3-4tsp of the Heal Thyself Master Herbal Formula to increase circulation

Action

Take 2-4 salt baths 3-4 times a week. Use 1-2lbs of *Epsom or Dead Sea salt or 1 cup apple cider vinegar

Take hot and cold showers daily

*Use apple cider vinegar if you have high blood pressure

Movement

Rebounding, jumping, swimming, and massaging to move the lymphatic system

Perform 30min -1 hour daily

EARTH ELEMENT TO REBUILD THE BODY

EARTH ELEMENT RULES THE BONES & COLON

EARTH THERAPHY for Optimal Wellness

The 4 Element Green Living Chart presents a systematic green-living way to restore the anatomy on the spiritual, emotional and physical levels by using plants. Reach optimal wellness using a plant based diet, daily ingest up to 1 pint of green juice. Add 1-2 Tbs. of Green Life Nutritional formula to green juice or H20.

Take Green Life & Green Juice for 2 consecutive weeks to break the cycle of chronic dis-ease.

The Heal Thyself Green Life Formula is a nutritiously sound compound that contains a full range of vitamins such as vitamin A, B complex, C , E, bio-flavo-noid, choline, essential fatty acids, selenium, inositol, plus minerals such as cal-cium , copper, iodine, magnesium, manganese, phosphorus, silicon, sodium, sulfur, and zinc. Green Life also contains wheatgrass, a soil based plant, and spirulina, a water based plant that will rejuvenate and detoxify.

Reasons for performing earth therapy:
This intensive system of rejuvenation will aid in establishing a skeletal struc-ture that is free of pain and a colon that is free of impacted waste; to nourish your body and to raise your frequency. Performing the suggested earth thera-pies also assists in overcoming rage, jealousy, verbal abuse, envy, selfishness, depression, procrastination, and desire to perform destructive sexual activities.

How to perform earth therapy:
Formula
Drink 2 - 3 8oz glasses of freshly pressed Green Juice with 1 Tbsp of Heal Thyself Green Life Nutritional Formula.

Action
Apply Heal Thyself Rejuvenation Clay treatment to areas of pain 2-4 times a week.

Movement
Biking, jogging, power walking, calisthenics, weight lifting, or drum-ming. Perform 30 min – 1 hour daily.

Recite
"May I be protected by 70 purifications I purify myself at the great stream of the galaxy, and that which is wrong in me is pardoned and the spots upon my body and upon the earth are washed away. I come that I may purify this soul of mine in the Most High Degree."

CHAPTER 4

MAN
HEAL THYSELF

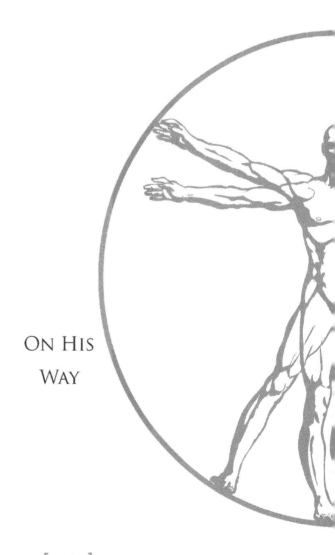

ON HIS
WAY

In this chapter, Man Heal Thyself, you are provided with the instructions for using the tools and strategies for wellness that are throughout the book. This is the workbook section of your text.

MAN HEAL THYSELF

MAN HEAL THYSELF. When you cannot see yourself and your eyes are in a haze, your mind is in a fog and you cannot find your way, I see you. Beyond your weaknesses, beyond your hurt, beyond your wounds, beyond your imperfections and shortcomings, I clearly see your greatness; your potential. I see your radiance and your beauty beyond the ugly and the shallow. I see your strength, your nobility. I see your efforts to climb out of the "barrel of crabs ". I see your dreams deferred and your hopes realized; your falls and your risings. I see you gasping for breath, and lost for words. I see your light at the end of the tunnel and your awesome possibilities.

MAN HEAL THYSELF. I see you as you are. When all else seems to fail, I know you will overcome, make it happen, break through the fog and haze; bring it home. I promise to hold a steady watch until you come into your own, raising your frequencies with your own hands. I light a candle at the window, keeping the faith that one day you will see what I see. From the first moment we hold you as a baby boy in our arms, we womenfolk pray for you. In our hearts we know you will grow great, marvelous and brilliant. We keep the faith.

I see you growing from an incomplete, wounded man of dis-ease to a Man Healing Thyself, and ultimately into a Supreme Man of Optimal Wellness. I see who you really are, from the depths of your despair to the heights of your wellness. I deem this as the time for men to take The Great Walk and Journey into your Holistic Wholeness. It is time for men to acknowledge and heed your inner wisdom. It is time for you to utilize the power in plants, earth, water, air, fire and spirit as the natural tools for your detoxification from dis-ease and your wellness restoration. I see man radiant again with the pure balanced power of the Optimal Wellness Man of the Emerald Age of Wellness.

MAN HEAL THYSELF. It is your time to learn the lessons that life offers you. Shed the pain, regret, anger and sorrow. Shed procrastination. Rise, now. Wherever you may be on your life path, dare to begin to rebirth yourself. Be who you really are. Dare to see what I see.

MEN HEAL THYELF. Since the Million Man March in 1995 many have died who could have lived. Others, who could have strengthened their limbs, are crippled; others, who could have been free, are spending life in prison. Those who are addicted to drugs, alcohol, cigarettes, fast and junk food could have detoxed and broken the cycle of addiction. Far too many have been physically and emotionally beating up themselves and their families because conditions in society have beaten them down. They could have been whole, living a life of harmony and balance. It is not too late.

I am calling a million to health. Whether you are a Christian man, a Muslim man, a Buddhist man, a Khamitic man, a Hebrew/Israelite man, an Atheist man, or a Universalist; whether you are a doctor or a blue- collar worker, you can Heal Thyself and move to a safe place; a higher ground.

I am calling a million men to rise up to wellness...to make a change. Now is your time, MAN HEAL THYSELF. Follow the road map from a man of disease and degeneration to a Man of Wellness. Become a Wellness Warrior of Power. Become a Heal Thyself Man of Vitality. Become a Supreme Man of Optimal Wellness. Man, be reminded of the words of the Honorable Marcus Garvey, "Up, up you mighty people, you can accomplish what you will."

It is indeed your time.

WHAT WE EAT

"We Are What We Eat"
HONORABLE ELIJAH MOHAMMAD

*"Food is not just vitamins and minerals, food it is spiritual.
Food seeks spirituality through us and we seek spirituality through the food."*
DR. LLAILA AFRIKA

What we eat creates who we are and what we become. It refers to all the things we take into our bodies, minds and spirits. With our bodies we eat the food, drink the water and breathe the air that is in our environment. Whether they are personal, social or business-related we ingest the relationships in our lives into our bodies, minds and spirits. We consume our whole living experience into our whole selves, whether you are Wounded Man or Wellness Man, your dis-eases or your state of wellness depends on what you consume. You are the sum total of all that you take into yourself. Figuratively and literally, "You are what you eat".

Food creates the body, builds the mind and liberates the spirit. The higher the frequency of food ingested the more vibrant and elevated Man becomes. As Man travels through the 12 States of Man he will learn to consciously choose the food he will in order to prevent dis-ease and obtain optimal benefits for wellness. Eating whole organic food creates whole men free of dis-ease.

DIETARY ENEMIES OF MAN

1. PROTEINS

FLESH:

pork, beef, goat, lamb, chicken, fish

RELATED DIS-EASES:

numbing sensation in the extremities; cancer: prostate, colon, throat, etc.; kidney failure, enlarged testicles, toxic sperm

DIETARY WELLNESS PROTEIN ALTERNATIVES:

TVP beans, lentils, sprouts, raw nuts and seeds, Heal Thyself Green Life Nutritional Formula

2. CARBOHYDRATES

CARBS:

White rice, white bread, white potatoes

DIS-EASE RELATED:

constipation, abdominal bloating, gas, shortness of breath

DIETARY WELLNESS CARB ALTERNATIVES:

sprouted bread, brown rice, couscous, bulgur wheat, tabouli, buck wheat pancakes

3. FATS/OIL

UNHEALTHY FATS/OIL:

polyunsaturated fats, trans-fats and saturated fats

RELATED DIS-EASES:

high blood pressure, strokes, numbness sensation, sluggishness

DIETARY WELLNESS FATS/OILS ALTERNATIVES:

Cold pressed olive oil, sesame oil, cold pressed flaxseed oil

4. CALCIUM

DAIRY:

Milk, cheese, ice cream, butter, eggs, yogurt, etc.

RELATED DIS-EASES:

constipation, clogged arteries, respiratory issues, blockage, asthma, colds, allergies, snoring, toxic/acidic sperm

DIETARY WELLNESS DAIRY ALTERNATIVES:

almond milk, sesame milk, green vegetable juice

5. SWEETS

SUGAR:

corn syrup, fructose, brown and white sugar

DIS-EASE RELATED:

Diabetes, stress, arthritis aches and pains, headaches, depressions, mood swings, devitalized weak sperm

DIETARY WELLNESS SWEET ALTERNATIVES:

licorice root, raw honey, dates, raisins, currents, agave, stevia

6. SALT

TABLE SALT:

Iodized Salt

RELATED DIS-EASES:

high blood pressure, stroke, impotency

DIETARY WELLNESS SALT ALTERNATIVES:

sea salt, kelp, dulse, and nori

7. INGESTIBLE ENEMIES OF MAN:

drugs, alcohol, cigarettes, soft drinks, coffee

RELATED DIS-EASES:

shortens life span, weakens immune system, damages the liver and lungs, devitalized weak sperm

WELLNESS ALTERNATIVES TO USING INGESTIBLE ENEMIES:
Invert body for 10 minutes, write in your Journal, Recite Man Heal Thyself Daily Declarations and Affirmations, Rise between 4AM and 5AM and Perform Manifestation Practice to integrate the wellness regime with the elements of your wellness (Air, Fire, Water, Earth)

OTHER DIETARY ENEMIES (THE PATHWAY TO AN IMPOTENT LIFE):
genetically engineered foods, microwave foods, fried foods, pasteurized foods, chemically saturated fruits, nuts, grains and beans

DIS-EASE RELATED:
chronic fatigue, numbing, mean spirited, hostile, depressed, devitalized weak sperm

WELLNESS ALTERNATIVES TO OTHER DIETARY ENEMIES:
incorporate holistic tools and strategies in your daily lifestyle. Follow the instructions provided on the Man Heal Thyself Scrolls (Charts).

SETTING UP YOUR NUTRITION KITCHEN HEALING LABORATORY

As you begin your a detox plan you should prepare your environment. Below are some things you may need to obtain in order to set up your kitchen as a laboratory for creating your wellness.

Items you will need to facilitate converting your kitchen into a Healing/ wellness laboratory:
    Juicer: to juice live fruits and vegetables
    Blender: to blend juices, sauces and nutrients
    Stainless steel pots: for preparing steam vegetables and herbal teas
    Charts (See products in the back of this book):
    The City of Wellness Nutrition Kitchen, Pyramids of Wellness

Also consider:

Food Processor: for preparing vegetables to make soups and salads

Dehydrator: for preparing Live Cookies, Croquettes, Pie Fillings, Veggie Chips

Sprouter: for growing your own Alfalfa Sprouts, Mung bean Sprouts, Broccoli Sprouts

---

As stated at the opening of this book, if you are presently consulting a physician for existing health challenges, CONTINUE to follow the advice of your physician. The information provided here is designed to be inspirational and help you make informed decisions about your health. This material is NOT intended to be a substitute for any medical advice or treatment that has been prescribed by your physician.

Use the tools in your kitchen laboratory and your charts (The City of Wellness Nutrition Kitchen and Pyramids of Wellness) to plan your meals. Consult your Man Heal Thyself Scroll to plan the rest of your holistic, each day of your Wellness Life.

These are basic steps or levels of food consumption. Most people's food plan exists on more than one of them. To detox and rejuvenate try to prepare, eat and drink one step higher than your present level. For optimal wellness follow the Advanced Juice Fast for 7 consecutive days as you travel on your 12 week journey.

WEEK 1 - 3
LEVEL 1 – BEGINNER – FLEXITARIAN

The Family Man | The Sensual Man | The Transformation Man

Consume vegetable protein as well as organic chicken and unshelled fish. Incorporate beans, peas, sprouts, and lentils into your diet. Omit all other flesh foods (beef, pork, lamb, turkey, goat, etc) Consume more fresh fruit, vegetables, and whole grains.

WEEK 4 - 6
LEVEL 2 – INTERMEDIATE – VEGETARIAN

The Lover Man | The Communication Man | The Intuitive Man

Consume only vegetarian foods, Omit all flesh foods (Seafood, beef, pork, lamb, turkey, goat, etc). Fresh vegetable intake includes 50% or 75% live food and 50% or 25% steamed to retain as much of the live enzymes and oxygen as possible.

WEEK 7-9
LEVEL 3 – ADVANCED VEGAN (RAW)

The Universal Man | The Illuminator Man | The Harmonizing Man

Consume 100% live, uncooked food. Live food include organic live proteins (sprouted beans, raw soaked nuts and seeds, avocados) , live soups , uncooked grains such as couscous, tabouli, bulgar wheat etc. Consume whole or juiced fresh fruits and vegetables. Drink daily warm water (8oz), 5 cups Herbal Master Tea and 8oz of Kidney- Liver Flush.

WEEK 10-12
LEVEL 4 – ADVANCED WHOLE FOOD
THERAPUTIC JUICE FAST

The Natural Man | The Alchemist Man | The Optimalist Man

Consume 100% organic liquid meals only. This cleansing level meal consists, daily, of two vegetable juice meals for rejuvenation and one fruit meal for detoxification. Additionally, there is a daily intake of ½ galoon warm water , 5 Cups Herbal Master Tea and 8oz of Kidney–Liver Flush every day. LEVEL 4 is a therapeutic juice fast that should be followed for (7) seven days each season (84 days) Elements of the juice fast are part of all four steps.

SETTING UP YOURSELF FOR THE MAN HEAL THYSELF JOURNEY

Prepare your mind.

Read material on wellness. Although your decision to detox is a private and individual one, for support, you may choose to speak to others who are on the path to becoming a Supreme Man of Optimal Wellness.

Prepare your spirit.

Consider reciting and reflecting upon the affirmations from the both the Teachings of Antiquity and the Heal Thyself affirmations. Choose and reflect upon words that are appropriate to the situation you want to restore to wellness or the body part member you are focusing on to revitalize and rejuvenate.

Prepare for and perform Man Heal Thyself Meditation and Vision Quest

Man Heal Thyself

Step 1

Early Morning Rise between 4 AM – 6 AM to maximize your soul's connection with your meditation and affirmations. Cleanse your internal body; drink (16 oz. warm water with juice of 1-2 lemons or limes).

Step 2

Cleanse your spiritual channel; quite your mind and spirit.

Step 3

Recite Man Heal Thyself Healing and Harmonizing Meditation (See Epigraph). For further suggestions of affirmations, also see in this chapter: I AM MAN.

Sit on a comfortable seat with back straight, shoulders down, chest open and place palms open. Close your eyes and go within your heart as you connect to your breath. Now inhale, as your chest and diaphragm expand and exhale as you release all tension and stress. After several inhalations and exhalations you will become centered and totally relaxed. Now that you're relaxed, travel with your mind and your breath to the body member that is in need of healing. Now inhale and exhale within the body member that you are working on transforming. After several times breathing in and out, a deep sense of Maát will emanate through the specific body part that you are working on. With each breath of renewal you will raise your frequency and come closer and closer to reaching optimal wellness.

Step 4 – Man Heal Thyself Vision Quest

Tap into your Vision Quest, and come into alignment with your higher consciousness. Be courageous, go within. Travel to unchartered territory. Stay within your breath, as you inhale ask the question and as you exhale listen for the answer about your work, of your mission. Listen for how to let go and how to embrace. Discover your purpose for being and how to arrive at your destination of greatness, of clarity, of peace. The vision may come loudly; it may even scream at you; or it may come in a whisper. Stay close, pay attention, listen, receive then watch for the miracle as your soul releases the treasures that are within your reach.

Step 5

Record the Findings of Your Vision Quest- Write about your meditation or vision quest in your journal. Write what guidance you received about your vision. Write the questions you still have and the plans you are making to accomplish your vision.

Step 6

Activate 'The Message'; Stay on your path to your vision. Trust your inner vision; follow the guidance, move on the message. Diligently build your life's work. Embrace the treasure; manifest your prosperity. Manifest a fulfilling and prosperous life. Breath deeper, open your eyes and Give Thanks.

A Man Heal Thyself Man builds bridges, builds homes; builds institutes; builds his body, mind and spirit.

BUILD YOUR VISION.
BUILD YOUR LIFE OF OPTIMAL WELLNESS.

I AM MAN

I AM A MAN is dedicated to Dr. Martin Luther King and the Honorable Malik Shabazz (Malcolm X). Each was an both extraordinary Optimal Man who fought, labored, marched, and spoke up for our freedom as a civil right! Optimal Freedom Is Wellness

SHOUT & AFFIRM YOUR FREEDOM DAILY

I am free from procrastination. I am empowered to move forward.	I am empowered to move forward.
I am free from violence.	I am empowered to be at peace.
I am free from poverty.	I am free to acquire prosperity.
I am free from stagnation.	I am free to move forward.
I am free from destruction.	I am free to build & create greatness.
I am free from hurt and disappointment.	I am free to forgive and be forgiven.
I am free from drug addiction.	I am free to live fully and be elevated on Green Life formula.
I am free from burdens.	I am free to release the weight of the world.
I am free from STD's.	I am empowered to live free of STD's.
I am free from premature aging.	I am empowered to reverse the aging process.
I am free from fast food addiction	I am empowered to embrace whole food living
I am free from couch potato-pot belly syndrome.	I am free to be mentally and physically sound and fit.
I am free from continuing to pass on toxic DNA	I am empowered to live dis-ease free.
I am free from stress.	I am to embrace a calm state of serenity

Prepare to record your journey to wellness.
Purchase or prepare a notebook to record your experiences of transformation to wellness of body, mind and spirit.

(Sample) Vision Quest Journal Page

Rise | Shine | Listen | Receive | Activate

(Put here: Date and Level of 12 States of Man you are on (Sample)

_____

_____

_____

_____

_____

_____

_____

_____

_____

_____

_____

_____

The Power To Heal Is Within

HOW TO USE THE MAN HEAL THYSELF SCROLL

The Man Heal Thyself Scroll is a road map, a guide on how to holistically and actively bring yourself to Wellness. Apply the work of the scroll to restore your body. The Man Heal Thyself Scrolls are located in Chapters with the Arit Stats of Man Heal Thyself. Added each week are strategies for use of food, meditation and body work. Remember your goal is to purify and restore all the parts of yourself. When you work to bring dynamic wellness and harmony to your whole anatomy: body, mind and spirit, you, Heal Thyself Man, can become like a concert of the richest sound.

Definitions of categories used on the Man Heal Thyself Scroll:

Anatomy of Man deals with the **total** anatomy. Focus on the body member at hand that you are working on to detoxify and rejuvenate. for 7 – 12 weeks and put behind the call out the Man Heal Thyself lifestyle and you will restore thyself. Daily remember that the power to heal is within.

Antiquity Affirmation

Meditate at sunrise and sunset, daily. Sit quietly and recite. The antiquity affirmation (or one you have chosen). As you speak, you become what you speak. Speak yourself into existence. Recite affirmations to awaken your "dry bones". Resurrect yourself with each word. The Antiquity Affirmations are all based on Nile Valley of KMT Healing Affirmation from the first civilization. Light a white candle and light up your heart. Allow the ancient ones, the shining beings, to shine through as you speak your body temple into wakefulness.

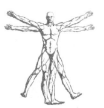

Metaphysical Charge/Physical Metaphysical Dis-Ease

Thoughts are things what we think in our mental body (mind) s and feel in our in our physical body and feel we create in our physical bodies. We can reshape our lives by the transformation of our mind. Each day speak through our words what you need to bring your body temple to wholeness to healing. Food Is Medicine

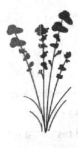

Herbal Compound

If you have a chronic dis-ease, for one to three week, take the specific herbal compound that supports the recovery of the specific body member. Boil 3 cups of water at night, turn off the flame and then add 3 teaspoons of each loose herbs. Cover pot and steep overnight. In the morning strain tea, then drink before noon.

Loose Herbs:

Steep 1 tsp of loose herbs in 1 cup of distilled water. Strain and drink

Powdered Herbs:

Steep ¼ tsp of herbal powder in 1 cup of distilled water. Strain and drink.

Tinctures:

Add 10 drops to 1 cup of distilled water. Strain and drink.

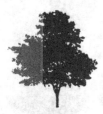

Nature Balms

Nurture yourself with nature by drinking your tonics. Bath yourself with Epsom salt or Apple Cider Vinegar or Master Herbal Tonic, then massage yourself with olive oil, castor oil or almond oil to bring harmony to the psychological, emotional and physical parts of your anatomy.

Clay Poultice

For three to seven weeks apply a 1" poultice (clay pack) over the areas of the body that are swollen, inflamed, or in pain. Cover the ends of the gauze with non-surgical tape to keep gauze in place. Leave the poultice on overnight. In the morning take a warm shower.

Zone Massage

There are reflexology points on the face, hand and feet that connect to the organs and systems, (respiratory, circulatory, etc,) of the body. Massaging of the reflexology points stimulates blood flow to the related body part member and or system.

MAN HEAL THYSELF DAILY CHECK- UP

Check off your progress on your path to Optimal Wellness.

Sunrise Wellness

	Day 1	Day 2	Day 3	Day 4	Day 5	Day 6	Day 7
Recite/Reflect on Affirmation from Antiquities and Heal Thyself							
Drink the juice of lemons and 16oz of warm water with 2 Tbsp colon base							
Invert body for 10 minutes							
Have Green Life Liquid Breakfast (8oz fresh juice with 8oz H2o +1-2 Tbsp of Green Life)							
Liquid Meal 30 minutes later Solid Meal							
Drink Master Herbal Formula							

Midday Wellness (Lunch)

	Day 1	Day 2	Day 3	Day 4	Day 5	Day 6	Day 7
Green Life Liquid Lunch (8-16 oz fresh juice or H2O with 1-2 Tbsp of Green Life)							

	Day 1	Day 2	Day 3	Day 4	Day 5	Day 6	Day7
Solid Lunch Vegan Lunch: Green Power Lunch (i.e., Salad/ steamed vegetables/ whole grains/veg- etable, protein, i.e. beans, lentils)							
Flexitarian Lunch: Steamed fish as pro- tein with vegetables and whole grains							

Sunset Wellness (Dinner)

	Day 1	Day 2	Day 3	Day 4	Day 5	Day 6	Day 7
Liquid Dinner Green Life Nutritional dinner (8-16 oz of vegetable juice and H2O with 1-2tbsp Green Life Nutri- tional Formula)							
Green Power Dinner (i.e., salad/steamed vegetables/whole grains/vegetables protein, i.e., beans, peas lentils)							
Flexitarian Dinner: Steamed fish as pro- tein with vegetables and whole grains							

	Day 1	Day 2	Day 3	Day 4	Day 5	Day 6	Day 7
Man Life Herbal Tonic (7days) alternate Master Herbal Tonic (7days). Directions: Add 6 tbsp to 4oz of boiling H2O and let steep for 1hr (off of the stove). Drink before bedtime.							
Take 3 Herbal Laxative Tablets							
Detox Bath Soak in warm water tub with 1-2lbs Epsom Salt. Soak for 30 minutes							
Zone Body Massage body, face, hands,							
Apply clay over the body member in need over night							

"HEALTH IS THE MOST IMPORTANT THING
THIS UNIVERSE HAS.

IT IS THE FIRST AND LAST
OF YOUR EXISTENCE OR EXISTING.

A WISE MAN HAS GOOD HEALTH
BECAUSE OF LOVE FOR THE BODY.

LOVE IS INJECTED
AND THEN PROJECTED.

SELF-LOVE SHAPED AND
SHAPES THE UNIVERSE."

DR. PAUL GOSS
AUTHOR OF: THE NATURAL WAY/ FOUNDER OF NEW BODY PRODUCTS

CHAPTER 5

MAN
HEAL THYSELF/
MAN OF VITALITY

THE FIRST 7 ARIT STATES OF MAN

Arit State 1:
The Family Man of Unity and Wealth

Arit State 2:
The Sensual Man of Heightened Sensitivity and Sexual Prowess

Arit State 3:
The Transformation Man of Renewal

Arit State 4:
The Lover Man of Harmony

Arit State 5:
The Communication Man of Sensitvity and Creatvity

Arit State 6:
The Intuitive Man of Inner Vision

Arit State 7:
The Universal Humanitarian Man

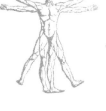
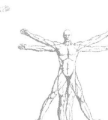

WHAT IS THE ARIT?

The arit or aritu (plural) are energy within the human body. They are the same as the chakra system[1], which can be represented as wheels of flowers or wheels of light. They are round and approximately 1 foot in diameter. When the body is vibrant and healthy, the aritu spin clockwise. When the body is toxic, the aritu spin counterclockwise. The arit is the spiritual center that communicates by sending messages and signals to the body. It is encoded with information about the lifetimes of one's being, essentially functioning like a reference library or a time capsule. The information is able to reach the physical and mental bodies according to the condition of the arit. The arit also functions like a lighthouse that radiates frequencies and electrical currents which register high or low, determining the frequency of the body, mind and spirit. If the arit energy is high one will enjoy optimal wellness. If the arit energy is low the individual will suffer from poor health. The arit contains within itself the masculine hemisphere of consciousness which rules material, intellectual and financial conditions. While the feminine consciousness rules the spiritual, creative and intuitive side of man. As one journeys through the 12 arit, or states of man, and applies Man Heal Thyself practices of meditation, affirmation, food is medicine, self-massage, breathing exercises, herbology and elemental healing (healing with earth, air, fire and water), man will bring himself into an optimal state of well-being.

---

[1]The arit and the chakras are one in the same. The arit is the original name that was born out of Afri-Khametic teachings, and the word chakra, as an extension of that, was born out of Hindu teachings.

"ARRANGE FOR ME THE WAY.
MAY I RENEW MYSELF.
MAY I BECOME STRONG."
FROM: PAPYRUS OF ANI

ALI'S STORY

I can illuminate the journey that all men must travel in order to heal themselves by sharing a little bit of my personal story. We all begin our journey long before coming into the womb, but I will start my story from the day I was born.

My mother, Queen Afua separated from my father when I was about 1 year old. For a while, she raised me, my brother and sister as a single mother. And then she remarried and my siblings and I enjoyed the benefits of having a father figure in our lives. Still, all of the feelings my mother felt as she went through her transitions with my father became neurologically imprinted on each of us in a slightly different way. I carried this imprint with me until eventually I met and grew deeply in love with a beautiful woman who would become my daughter's mother. Our relationship was sweet, but eventually it turned out to be as volatile as it was passionate. The love we felt for each other was intense. And when we expressed a vibration other than love, it was equally as intense. We fought bitterly and vacillated back and forth between joy and pain for a while. Somewhere in between that time we got engaged and conceived our daughter, Maatia, in the fullest expression of love. But eventually the volatility took over and she and I separated. Although I had known many people who were, in one way or another, products of a broken family, I was unprepared for what happened next. My ex took my daughter away from me, and I don't mean she moved out to another neighborhood or city, even. For two and a half years I had no idea where Maatia was. It was like my baby had been kidnapped. I was desperate to find my child because I missed her so, and perhaps, more importantly, something deep inside me knew that she needed me as much as I needed her. I knew, intuitively, that if I didn't use all my heavenly and earthly resources to find her that it could seriously damage, or destroy her. Even if I couldn't find her, I needed to be able to tell her, one day, if that day ever came, that I did everything in my power to reconnect with her. This is where the real challenge began. It was definitely hard to have lost track of my daughter, but it was even harder to find the courage to commit to finding her.

There are so many obstacles put before fathers who want to care for their children after their relationship with the child's mother ends. Those obstacles can be legal, financial, physical, mental, emotional, cultural, social, psychological, and/or spiritual. Usually it's a complex combination of all of these. I had to deal with an internal tug-of-war in which voices inside me and outside of me were telling me this was a lost cause, that my ex would be filling my daughter's head with hateful ideas about me and there would be nothing I could do about it, that I should stop stressing myself out, and that I had done enough at some point, and the rest would not be worth the trouble. On the other hand I knew I didn't want to set my daughter up for the inevitable lifelong struggle for self-worth that typically ensues when a father abandons his child. There are bruised and wounded daughters all over the world who attract a cycle of abusive relationships because they never got the chance to be "Daddy's Little Girl." I didn't want that fate to befall my child. I wanted to neurologically re-imprint her, so that she could know that I loved her and I wanted her, and so she could grow up to be healthy and whole and forge meaningful, loving relationships of her own. For two and a half years I had to fight through all of those different challenges as I engaged in a serious prolonged period of self-reflection and discovery. During that time, I discovered my true power.

I thought I was searching for Maatia because I wanted to save my daughter. The person I wound up saving was me.

For two years I trained myself to let go of my ego and my anger by meditating, consistently cleansing, surrounding myself with a council of elders (including a lawyer), and practicing gratitude for all the blessings I already had. I used the power of my mind to practice, for the day we would meet again, being non-reactionary, non-judgmental, and disciplined. I knew that if Maatia's mother and I saw each other again, it would be really easy for me to become undone. She could push my buttons, and she and I both knew it. I had to learn to "turn the other cheek"* and stay focused on my goal in order to heal myself and my daughter. I had to hire a private investigator who finally tracked down both of them. They were in New Orleans. (I was living in

New York at the time). We proceeded to go to court. The judge's ruling was that I could spend 4 hours, once a month with Maatia, in New Orleans, at my own expense. I was happy to have found Maatia, and at the same time, I was devastated that after all of my hard work, this measly visitation arrangement was the outcome. I could hardly believe it. But I counted my blessings, and I held onto my peace of mind and peace of behavior.

In the ensuing months, I had incredibly trying conversations with my daughter's mother, and I even received hateful text messages from her mate, but I held onto my peace. (I also kept a record of all correspondence just in case there would be a need to present them in court in the future.) To keep myself grounded, I often repeated mantras like, "Breathe, receive, walk away, Ali." My ex fiancé was over an hour late bringing Maatia to our first visitation. "Breathe, receive, walk away Ali." I started to argue with her about it. For a minute, I got caught up in the ego trap. But I reminded myself to "Breathe, receive, walk away Ali." I smiled at my daughter with all the sincerity I could muster. I was so moved that she remembered me. After all, she was still a baby the last time I saw her, and now, she was 4 years old. She said to me, "You're handsome." I melted. I told her I had dreamed of her. She said she dreamed of me too. And somehow I knew that my struggle had not been in vain.

The most triumphant part of this story is yet to be told, because it is still unrevealed. There is much more for me to learn. But a sure sign that I have grown tremendously along this journey is that my ex and I have engaged in productive, harmonious conversations again. I have become an alchemist; one who transmutes the behavior of others around him, by first changing himself. I learned to trust my intuition. Yes, men have intuition too. I learned to be a better communicator, on the physical, mental and ethereal planes.

Queen has always said, "The power to heal is from within." We cannot force others to behave in a particular way in order to make us happy. In fact, it is their "mis-behavior" that often causes us to activate our own power to heal and grow. Although I have the rest of my life to spend loving Maatia, I've already become a greater father than I was before. I cherish every moment with her, and I make sure to create happy feelings and memories that she can pass along to her children. I am creating a legacy of wellness in my family by healing myself.

*Contrary to popular belief, the expression "turn the other cheek" requires a higher form of consciousness rather than a lesser form of reactionary behavior. It means to stay focused on "the prize" in spite of how reality may seem. It promotes looking consistently at what you *do* want, rather than what you *don't* want; no matter what.

THE FAMILY MAN OF UNITY & WEALTH
ARIT 1

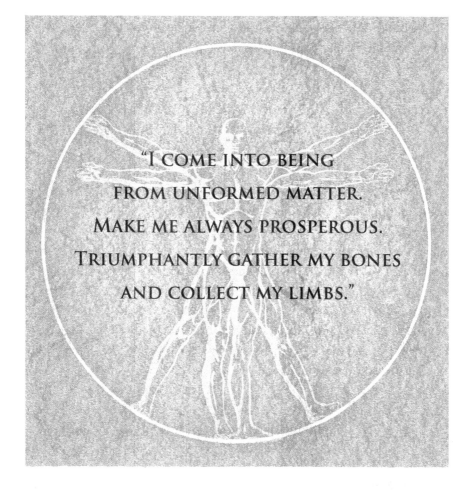

"I COME INTO BEING
FROM UNFORMED MATTER.
MAKE ME ALWAYS PROSPEROUS.
TRIUMPHANTLY GATHER MY BONES
AND COLLECT MY LIMBS."

A Family Man represents unity. Unity represents harmony and harmony creates abundance. Poverty is the result of discord. For one to be a Family Man, he must establish an inner state of unity. As a man unifies his inner self, his family reflects his inner harmony. The Family Man makes every possible effort to secure himself, and his family's survival with food, clothin, and shelter. His world revolves around building family, but nurturing family, communication with family and cultivating family.

The Family Man knows that family is the foundation and the root of his success. The Family Man's focus is to build material abundance in order to stabilize the unity and growth of the family.

The Family Man must possess creativitym visionm andan unwavering inner commitment to manifest a strong family.

COCCYGEAL ROOT EMPOWERMENT & DETOX AFFIRMATION

1ST ARIT

Affirm: My life is abundantly full and it is overflowing with greatness. May I be empowered to overcome financial lack. May I attract and build prosperity in all ways and may financial abundance flow like a river. May I create work that reflects my purpose. May I not abuse family, may I not be abused by my family. May I work with my family to build a powerful self-sustaining unit that supplies all our needs. May I, as a man bring to my family unity, power, and strength, that we not only survive but that we, as a family, thrives. Today, I attract not poverty, but wealth. I vibrate at the frequency of red which represents power and vitality, which as I heal my family I bring power and vitality to them. May my family honor and care for me.

WEEK 1 - THE FAMILY MAN OF UNITY & WEALTH

The Family Man dwells in the redroot coccygeal power center that houses the skin, legs & feet, muscular system and Bones.

Statistics: Arthritic men are 17.1 million of the people who have doctor-diagnosed arthritis. Half of the Americans with arthritis don't think anything can be done to help them. 4.6 million. Non-Hispanic Blacks report doctor diagnosed arthritis.

Anatomy of Man	Antiquity Affirmation	Metaphysical Wellness Charge	Physical Disease
I am a shining being. I have been created by and have come into existence from The Most High"	"I speak that I wish to become strong and it comes into being as I speak"	"Arrange for me the ways. May I renew myself. May I become strong."	"Arrange for me the ways. May I renew myself. May I become strong."
Skin Meditate and breathe deeply as you fill your skin with the light of purity.	"May I see my beauty. May I advance upon the Earth. Tehuti (Divine inner intelligence) Protects my flesh entirely."	**Metaphysical Dis-ease** Rage, resentment and anger **Power Charge** "I release all pinned up emotions that cause dis-ease."	**Physical Dis-ease** Eczema, black heads, shingles, boils
Legs and Feet Meditate and breathe deeply as you fill your legs and feet with the light of the full moon.	"Make strong my legs to rise up for me. I have gained power over my feet. May I stretch my feet which are fastened together."	**Metaphysical Dis-ease** Inability to move forward and to learn from lessons. **Power Charge** "I am free to move to higher ground"	**Physical Dis-ease** Water retention, swollen legs, feet and ankles
Muscular System Meditate and breathe deeply as you fill your muscular system with the light of strength.	"I shall not be seized by my arms, nor shall I be carried away by my hands, nor shall I allow anyone to bring harm to me."	**Metaphysical Dis-ease** Lack of self-control **Power Charge** "I am strengthened through every challenge."	**Physical Dis-ease** Sore aching muscles
Bones Meditate and breathe deeply as you fill your bones with hope.	"I come into being from unformed matter. Make me always prosperous. Triumphantly gather my bones and collect my limbs."	**Metaphysical Dis-ease** Fearful of the unknown shattered dreams, broken vision **Power Charge** I move in strength	**Physical Dis-ease** Arthritis, tooth decay, swollen joints

Herbal Compound	Nature Balm	Clay Poultice	Zone Massage
"I come into being from unformed matter. I grow into the form of plants."	"An ounce of prevention is worth a pound of cure."	"In the beginning The Most High gave every people a cup of clay and they drank their life." From Proverbs of Digger Indians	"I am the knot within the olive tree."
Aloe, Burdock, Sarsaparilla Drink herbal tea and herbal bath	Mix equal parts of organic oatmeal and cornmeal with water and scrub skin with loofa brush. Then wash and shower.	Apply Heal Thyself Rejuvenation Clay over skin and let air dry for 1 hour. Take a bath and add 1-2lbs of salt or apple cider vinegar (if you have high blood pressure)	**Face:** Massage the jawbones on both sides of the face. **Hands:** Massage the padding of each hand. **Feet:** Massage the heels of each foot.
Massage with Arnica Cream, Wintergreen Oil, or birch Feet: Full foot massage.	Increase vegetable protein (i.e. beans, lentils, soaked nuts, etc.) Add 1 Tbsp of Green Life Nutritional Formula to 8-12oz of distilled water and drink 3 times a day.	Apply Heal Thyself Rejuvenation Clay to gauze and place over legs and feet where there is pain and leave on overnight. Take a warm shower in the morning. Complete this process 3 times a week.	**Hands:** Full hand massage. **Feet:** Full foot massage.
Bonset, Horsetail, Yucca, Alfalfa	Juice ½ cup of fresh turnips with 8oz. of dark vegetable juice.	Apply Heal Thyself Rejuvenation Clay to guaze and place over painful bones and joints and leave on over night. Take a shower in the morning and wash from body. Complete this process at least 3 times a week	**Face:** Massage jaw bones for general stimulation. **Hands:** Massage fingers on both hands for general stimulation. **Feet:** Massage toes on both feet for general stimulation.

NUTRITION KITCHEN PHARMACY

*"In the midst of its streets and on either side of the river, was the tree of life,
which bore 12 fruits, each tree yielding its fruit every month. And the leaves of
the tree were for the healing of the nations. "*

REVELATION 22:2

Level 1 – Beginner – Flexitarian or Vegetarian Week 1 – 1st 21 Days

Consume vegetable protein as well as organic chicken and unshelled fish. In corporate beans, peas, sprouts, and lentils into your diet. Omit all other flesh foods (beef, pork, lamb, turkey, goat etc.) Consume more fresh fruits, vegetables and other whole grains.

Week 1 – The Family Man   Week 2 – The Sensual Man
Week 3 – The Transformation Man

Pre- Breakfast (Liquid)	Kidney Liver Flush Juice**:of 1 lemon, (if no HBP) 1 pinch of cayenne pepper, 1-2T Inner-Colon Ease
	8 oz. of warm water w/1-2 garlic cloves or 12 drops of kyolic
	Tool: Blender
Liquid Breakfast 7:00	8-12oz. Orange juice w/1-2T Green Life 12-16oz distilled water before
	BF=Breakfast (Master Herbal Tea or Woman's Life Tea)**
Solid Breakfast 7:30	1-2 Mangos or cantaloupe slices from one whole cantaloupe.
	*30 minute break between Eating & Drinking.
	*Optional Whole Grain Cereal with Almond or Sesame Milk

Liquid Lunch 12:00	Kale ½ cup, string beans ½ cup Cabbage ½ cup Add 1-2 T Green Life Formula Wheatgrass 1-2 or 3-7 times a week with 12-16oz of H2o Tool: Juicer
Solid Lunch 12:30	50% Salad Live Greens Asparagus w/ Dandelion Greens 30% Steamed Veggies Mustard Greens w/pearl onions or Vegetable Broth or Vegetable soup. 10%-20% Starch Soaked couscous w/ sunflower seeds & spike seasonings 10%-20% Protein or baked organic chicken (remove skin) Organic BBQ Tofu & Cajun seasonings ..... Eat animal protein midday only or steam unshelled fish
Liquid Dinner 6:00	Repeat lunch vegetable juice, and add 1-2 T Green Life 12-16oz water
Solid Dinner 6:30	50% Salad Live Greens: Escarole, kale w/ red pepper 30% steamed veggies: curry cauliflower 10%-20% Starch: Millet 10%-20% Vegan protein *When sun goes down, do not eat proteins or starches. Eat only fruits & salads.* 30 Min break between eating & drinking for optimal digestion of meal

Vision Quest Journal Page

Rise | Shine | Listen | Receive | Activate

Week 1 - The Family Man of Unity & Wealth

_____

_____

_____

_____

_____

_____

_____

_____

_____

_____

_____

_____

_____

_____

_____

_____

_____

_____

_____

_____

_____

The Power To Heal Is Within

THE SENSUAL MAN
OF HEIGHTENED SENSITIVITY

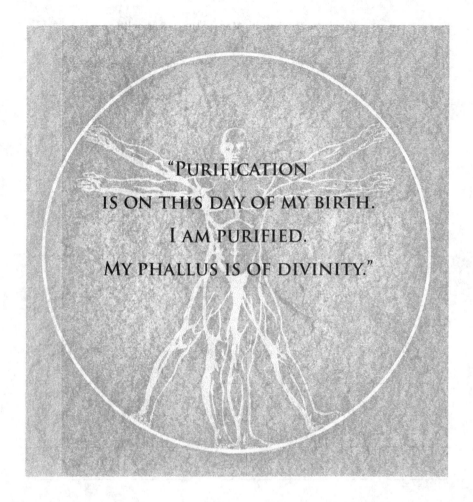

"PURIFICATION
IS ON THIS DAY OF MY BIRTH.
I AM PURIFIED.
MY PHALLUS IS OF DIVINITY."

ARIT 2

The Sensual Man is in tune with all of his senses; his visual sight, his inner-sight, his taste, his smell, and his touch, and is thus alive and aware of self and of the woman in his life, and life in general.

The Sensual Man is firm in body, steady in dispositions, and warm of heart. The sensual Man will hear your very thoughts. He will be intimate, sensitive, and connected to your every move. The sensual Man knows when to be still and when and how to approach. The Sensual Man is in harmony with his masculine and feminine balance. The Sensual Man's genitals are in their prime due to the total vibrant flow of blood and oxygen derived from a vegetable based lifestyle of Man Heal Thyself; which gives Man a potent, sensual sex life. The Sensual Man conceives and manifests healthy visions and children and/or worlds.

SACRED REPRODUCTIVE EMPOWERMENT AFFIRMATION

2ND ARIT

May my sacral center which houses my prostate, colon and bladder function in optimal wellness. Divine Healer within, may I bring forth life and strength in all I conceive, produce, and generate. May I gain and maintain power and vitality. May I maintain my youthful sexual and sensual creative life force. May I protect and guide my genitals from toxic thoughts, toxic emotions, toxic substances, and toxic relationships that keep me in a cycle of pain, conflict and constipation blockage. May my organs of release, i.e., colon and bladder support the purification of my entire anatomy so that I will draw to myself holistically healthy relationships.

WEEK 2 - THE SENSUAL MAN OF HEIGHTENED SENSITIVITY

The Sensual Man dwells in the prostate, bladder, colon and kidneys.

Statistics: Prostate – African American men have higher rates of getting and dying from prostate cancer than men of other racial or ethnic groups in the United States. http://www.medscape.com/viewarticle/497924

Anatomy of Man	Antiquity Affirmation	Metaphysical Wellness Charge	Physical Disease
I am a shining being. I have been created by and have come into existence from The Most High"	"I speak that I wish to become strong and it comes into being as I speak"	"Arrange for me the ways. May I renew myself. May I become strong."	"Arrange for me the ways. May I renew myself. May I become strong."
Prostate Meditate and breathe deeply as you fill your prostate with courage.	"Purification is on this day of my birth. I am purified. My phallus is of divinity"	**Metaphysical Dis-ease** Loss of self-esteem socio-economic pressure, lack of creativity **Power Charge** I am confident, potent & powerful	**Physical Dis-ease** STD's herpes, impotency, enlarged gonads
Bladder Meditate and breathe deeply as you fill your bladder with the light of confidence.	"I have created myself with Nu (water) in the name of Khepra." (trans-formation)	**Metaphysical Dis-ease** Feeling drained and out of control **Power Charge** "I am in control of my life."	**Physical Dis-ease** Weak and leaky bladder
Colon Meditate and breathe deeply as you fill your colon with the light of freedom.	"I have destroyed my inner enemies. I have removed my defects. My hindered parts are cleansed. I am pure coming forth by day."	**Metaphysical Dis-ease** Overwhelmed and filled with worry **Power Charge** "I am free of toxicity."	**Physical Dis-ease** Constipation distended abdomen
Kidneys Meditate and breathe deeply as you fill your kidneys with starlight.	"My kidneys are of Kheraba, a region of defense. I come forth from the water floods, given my inundations I gained from the River Nile."	**Metaphysical Dis-ease** Emotionally backed up. **Power Charge** "I am emotionally balanced and fortified.	**Physical Dis-ease** Edema, kidney failure, swelling

Herbal Compound	Nature Balm	Clay Poultice	Zone Massage
"I come into being from unformed matter. I grow into the form of plants."	"An ounce of prevention is worth a pound of cure."	"In the beginning The Most High gave every people a cup of clay and they drank their life." From Proverbs of Digger Indians	"I am the knot within the olive tree."
Cranberries, Blueberries, Raspberries, etc.	Apply Heal Thyself Rejuvenation Clay gauze and place over the kidneys and leave on overnight. Take a warm shower in the morning. Complete this process 3 times a week.	Blend 1 Tbsp of Heal Thyself Rejuvenation Clay with 8oz distilled water and drink 3-4 times a week.	**Face:** Use 3 fingers to massage from the face into the scalp. **Hands:** Massage the bottom of the palm of each hand. **Feet:** Use 4 fingers to massage from the front to the heel of each foot.
Cornsilk, Horsetail, Juniper, Uva Ursi	1 cup of fresh string beans and 1 clove of garlic and drink 4-5 times a day.	Blend 1 Tbsp of Heal Thyself Rejuvenation Clay with 8oz distilled water and drink 3-4 times a week.	**Hands:** Massage the center to palm of each hand. **Feet:** Massage the arch of each foot.
1 cup of okra 3-4 times a week, raw or steamed salad.	Take 3 Heal Thyself Herbal Laxatives with 16oz of warm water 3-4 times a week.	Apply Heal Thyself Rejuvenation Clay to gauze and place over abdomen and leave on overnight. Take a warm shower in the morning.	**Face:** Massage the cheeks bones on both sides of the face. **Hands:** Massage bottom of each thumb padding. **Feet:** Massage entire arch area of each foot.
Chickweed, Bladder Wrack, Fennel	Low vegetable protein such as cucumbers, ½ bunch of parsley, ½ bunch of watercress	Apply Heal Thyself Rejuvenation Clay to gauze and place over the kidneys and leave on overnight. Take a warm shower in the morning. Complete this process 3 times a week.	Face: Massage under each eye. Hands: Massage the padding of each hand. Feet: Massage the heels of each foot

Vision Quest Journal Page

Rise | Shine | Listen | Receive | Activate

Week 2 - The Sensual Man of Heightened Sensitivity

_____

_____

_____

_____

_____

_____

_____

_____

_____

_____

_____

_____

_____

_____

The Power To Heal Is Within

THE TRANSFORMATION MAN OF RENEWAL
ARIT 3

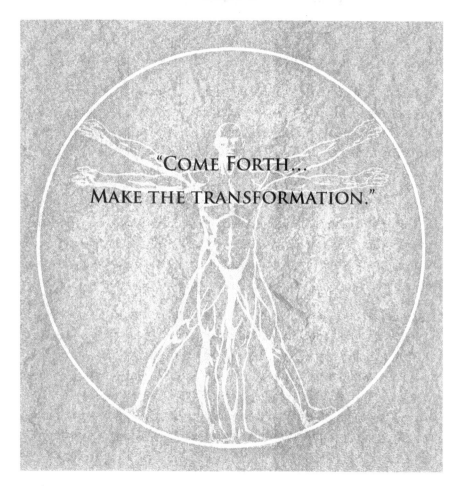

"COME FORTH...
MAKE THE TRANSFORMATION."

TRANSFORMATION OF MAN/
TRANSFORMATION OF THE EARTH

To the men from my clan, who are statistically the most traumatized from 400 years of chattel slavery, but who are most elevated as the first healers on Earth, I'm reaching out to you. Those who suffered as a casualty of a stolen legacy and who still suffer from the highest incidences of all dis-ease including economic starvation, emotional and psychological deprivation, and dietary malnutrition, I'm reaching out to you. To those suffering from the highest incidence of diabetes, high blood pressure, stroke, heart dis-ease, kidney failure, impotency, depression and premature death, I'm especially reaching out to you, to overcome, rise up and be counted in wellness. For YOU, the 1st man of humanity, this is your time.

Man, it's time to make a global shift from using power that destroys to using power that builds. For, power that destroys--and in these times especially--creates, massive, un-relentless dis-ease, greed, violence and wide spread destruction to nature and to Man. This is reflected and expressed through domination, suppression, oppression and manipulation.

Power that builds is True Power. It yields inner harmony, optimal health and balanced wealth. The Ancient Nile Valley ancestors called this state Maat (balance, truth, righteousness and reciprocity). As one applies the teachings in Man Heal Thyself, one comes into alignment. Man will draw to himself like a magnet, abundance in thought, word, and deed—and blossom, he will.

Through Man's mental, physical, emotional, social, and sexual elevation, he will shift the current conditions on Earth from toxic people, land, and environment, to holistic people who will restore the Earth. "As above, so below; as within, so without." Man's elevation will cause the air and water to purify and the Earth to recover in minerals and mass. Each day that Man grows in wellness, he will blossom and shift from an impotent, confused, weak, unsure, ineffective man, to a potent, empowered, healthy, vibrant, effective man.

In the beginning of time, Man was looked upon as Nefer-Atum, a Lotus Man in his illuminated state. Man has since fallen from his original way and is sometimes called the 'Old Dirty Bastard', so disease and violence covers the Earth.

Man needs a new day and a new way for a new earth to rise. Over the coming days, weeks, and seasons, Man will Heal Thyself through the Wellness protocols and they will bring Man to his full bloom as he awakens the Healer within. For the power to heal is within.

THE TRANSFORMATION MAN OF RENEWAL
ARIT 3

The Transformation Man has the ability to learn from every life experience. Through the process of Step One: Ingesting the Experience (recovering from the experience), and Step Two: Processing the Experience (living and digesting the experience). If the experience is for you, meaning it's part of your life force, then you become one with the experience and you grow with and through it. If the experience is indigestible and it is not meant for your development, then you as a Transformation Man, have the ability through detoxification, to learn from the experience which supports the Transformation Man to release the challenge, and the experience, to flush out the storm through prayer, meditation, visualization, journaling, healing baths, and soul sweats.

The Transformation Man is able to learn from every experience to grow, expand, and rise up from. The Transformation Man believes that every life lesson is a blessing.

"Transformation to higher ground – Transformation to a higher place"
KATRIEL WISE, THE MYSTIC MAESTRO

SOLAR PLEXUS EMPOWERMENT AFFIRMATIVE
3RD ARIT

May my solar plexus center, which houses my pancreas, liver, and kidney, function in optimal wellness. May I grow from all my experiences and come into a greater awareness of my power. May I assimilate, digest and release fully so that I may be elevated beyond excess. May I not be bound up with toxicity due to my challenging life experiences. May I receive a clear understanding of what I create so that I may grow abundantly throughout my life.

WEEK 3 - THE TRANSFORMATION MAN OF RENEWAL

The Transformation of Man metaphysically dwells in the Solar Plexus that houses the kidneys, liver, pancreas, and back.

Statistics: Diabetes is the leading cause of kidney failure in African American s. The prevalence of diabetes in African Americans is much higher than in white Americans. Approximately 14.7 percent of all African Americans over 20 years of age (3.7 million) have diabetes. On average, African Americans are twice as likely to have diabetes as white Americans if similar age. http://specturm.diabetesjournals.org/content/17/4/206.full

Pancreas: 13.0 million, or 11.8% of all men aged 20 years or older have diabetes.

Anatomy of Man	Antiquity Affirmation	Metaphysical Wellness Charge	Physical Disease
I am a shining being. I have been created by and have come into existence from The Most High"	"I speak that I wish to become strong and it comes into being as I speak"	"Arrange for me the ways. May I renew myself. May I become strong."	"Arrange for me the ways. May I renew myself. May I become strong."
Liver Meditate and breathe deeply as you fill your prostate with courage.	"Wisdom protects my flesh entirely"	**Metaphysical Dis-ease** Unresolved issues, feeling as if life's traumas are eating away at your organ.	**Physical Dis-ease** Cirrhosis of the liver
Pancreas Meditate and breathe deeply as you fill your pancreas with the light of conviction.	"Come Forth... Make the transformation".	**Metaphysical Dis-ease** Relationship breakdown **Power Charge** "I am whole for I am living a holistic life self & all my relations".	**Physical Dis-ease** Diabetes, loss of vision, amputation
Back Meditate and breathe deeply as you fill your back with the light of your path.	"My back is of vital power."	**Metaphysical Dis-ease** Lack of support from family, friends, and associates. **Power Charge** "I am supported in all areas of my life as I support life."	**Physical Dis-ease** Pain in the upper, middle and lower areas of the back

Herbal Compound	Nature Balm	Clay Poultice	Zone Massage
"I come into being from unformed matter. I grow into the form of plants."	"An ounce of prevention is worth a pound of cure."	"In the beginning The Most High gave every people a cup of clay and they drank their life." From Proverbs of Digger Indians	"I am the knot within the olive tree."
Physical Dis-ease	Omega fatty acids, safflower oil, 8oz. of 100% grapefruit juice 5 times a week, ½ cup of Jerusalem Artichoke juiced with 16 oz of dark green vegetables	Blend 1 Tbsp of Heal Thyself Rejuvenation Clay with 8oz distilled water and drink 3-4 times a week.	**Face:** Massage the side of the center of each ear. **Feet:** Massage under the center of the arch of each foot.
Blueberry Leaves, Marshmallow Agrimony, Burdock Root	1 cup of fresh string beans and 1 clove of garlic and drink 4-5 times a day.	Blend 1 Tbsp of Heal Thyself Rejuvenation Clay with 8oz distilled water and drink 3-4 times a week.	**Face:** Massage the jawbones on both sides of the face. **Hands:** Massage the padding of each hand. **Feet:** Massage the heels of each foot.
Dandelion and Alfalfa	Juice ½ cup of turnips, 4oz of kale and 4oz of chard and drink.	Apply Heal Thyself Rejuvenation Clay to gauze and place over spine and leave on overnight. Take a warm shower in the morning. Complete this process 3 times a week.	Face: Massage each jawbone. Hands: Massage the padding of each hand. Feet: Massage the heels of each foot

Vision Quest Journal Page

Rise | Shine | Listen | Receive | Activate

Week 3 - The Transformation Man of Renewal

_____

_____

_____

_____

_____

_____

_____

_____

_____

_____

_____

_____

_____

_____

_____

_____

_____

_____

_____

_____

_____

_____

The Power To Heal Is Within

THE LOVER MAN OF HARMONY
ARIT 4

"I AM PURE OF HEART
WITHIN A PURE BODY.
I EXIST IN MY HEART.
MAY MY HEART NOT BE TAKEN FROM ME.
LET IT NOT BE WOUNDED...
I KNOW MY HEART.
I HAVE GAINED POWER
OVER MY HEART."

LOVING OURSELVES; LOVING YOU

Just when I thought I was finished writing this book, *Man Heal Thyself*,
I attended a women's creative/political event. In the late evening, after a
very long day, I took a cab from Brooklyn to Harlem – I had been invited by a

sister- friend and I had to get there to show my support for the women pre-
senting the event. I jumped out of the cab and hurried through a steady rain
into a crowded, dimly lit room. Women, Black and of all races and political
orientations; women, wounded were in attendance in the room and express-
ing their feelings.

I was familiar with this room; I have been in rooms like this most of my
life. It was my mother's kitchen, my girlfriend's living room, my auntie's din-
ing room. In those rooms women talk about you: the men we used to love;
the one we love now; the men we want to love; the men we are done loving.
Sometimes it's so deep that we try to talk the love away just to stop the pain
of loving. In the room this rainy Friday night there was a circle of women and
a few men who cared to be there. Upon entering, I paused; I could feel what
was there and what was to come. It was on the walls and in the air. I almost
could not breathe as I was pulled into the heart of the room where women
were talking out loud, with hard beating breaths --about you. Woman
after woman took center stage and "ripped off her skin" in front of herself
and her sisters and the men who had cared to be there and were listening.
Poetically, courageously, the women revealed their hidden rage. Each one
shouted, screamed, wept, moaned and hollered to release the pain she had
kept silenced for too long. Her sisters and the men who had cared to be there
watched on.

Some of these women were running to the man in hopes that this time
it would be different from the last time. Others were running from lovers,
husbands, friends, partners; running for their lives. They had become afraid
of themselves in the state of unresolved fear that they saw reflected on your
face. Untreated fear had converted into rage…and the rage had converted
into war. The Gender War. Man against woman and woman against man, the
Gender War is swords pressed into each other until we bleed. It is women
thrusting angry faces; it is deep-seated, heart-bursting anger. It is generations
of pain. In the room artists, poets, dancers expressed the back-breaking madness of the Gender War with pulsating sounds, body-beating dance movements and words that thundered like stomping feet and bass drums. They

hit the floor with bare-fisted protests against the ongoing pain of unhealthy unions. They held their limbs in deformed positions to express, "Loving him hurts so bad, I'm feeling sad and broken." Their songs and dances said, "Man/ Woman, loving is natural but we have been so overexposed to the unnatural that we would rather maim and kill with looks and attitudes and words than be in pain in the name of love.

We women want to love you real good, but literally and figuratively we have been beaten and raped in the name of politics, social justice, and economics; and even in the name of love. Bad lovin' has wounded our hearts, attacked our wombs and made us...mad. "That's enough!" the women were saying in their poems and dances that night.

Man, Heal Thyself. Listen to the women as they tell we tell what is hurting us. You can't heal you, if you can't hear us; if you don't even don't listen to us. I am you; and you are me. We are the reflection of each other What I cre- ate is equally your creation. Such are the natural laws of Gender Peace.

So, just when I thought I was finished writing this book, *Man Heal Thyself,* I went to a women's event. They were in a room talking about themselves and about you. And because I am the Velvet Sword, and because this book is about men healing themselves, I had to write this article and tell you what we women are saying and thinking and feeling about loving ourselves, while loving you...

"There's a mystic seed that grows through a space that no one knows in the heart of Man. It nourishes the soul if allowed to unfold in the heart of Man."
LADY PREMA-CRYSTAL SAGE WOMAN

THE LOVER MAN OF HARMONY
ARIT 4

The true lover man is not a womanizer, a rolling stone, or a heart breaker. The lover man is filled with the pure spirit of the Most High. He has a huge heart filled with love, mercy, compassion and forgiveness...

The lover man heals the broken heart of wounded souls. A lover man honors and respects, restores not damages, and is trust worthy rather than dishonest. A lover man is not a double talker, he says what he means and means what he says. You can trust him with your heart.

The Lover Man fills the world with music, poetry, song, and dance with every thought, word, and deed. He pours love into the air. In the body of Lover Man there exists a safe haven – a place in him that you can trust to be honest. The Lover Man will nourish you mentally, emotionally, spiritually, and sexually. Even when at your worse state, one cannot take away from The Lover Man because his love is self-generating like the SUN.

The Lover Man carries within him a fiery heart that dissolves the rage of a fibroid tumor, a wounded heart that is seeking to be whole, or a broken spirit that needs mending. The touch of The Lover Man makes the coldest soul warm again. The Lover Man is his own Healer and he can heal himself leaving him free of heart dis-ease and strokes. A Lover Man of Soul Beauty will mystically bring you into a harmony profound.

HEART THYMUS EMPOWERMENT AFFIRMATION

4TH ARIT

May my heart center, which houses my blood stream, nervous system, circulatory system, lungs, back and core, function in optimal wellness. May my heart be not imbalanced, wounded and heavy. May my heart be in Maat (balanced harmonious forgiveness). With each life experience, may I breathe deep and full breaths in all that I do. May all my relations be renewed through my healthy heart. May I release from my heart burdensome relations as I learn from each lesson. May my heart be free of heart palpitations, heart attacks, and heart murmurs. May my healthy thoughts travel into my heart and help me to maintain a huge heart of mercy and compassion for myself and all my relationships.

WEEK 4 - THE LOVER MAN OF HARMONY

The Lover Man of Harmony dwells in the Green Heart Center that houses the nervous system, bloodstream, heart, and

Statistics: Nervous System – Among African Americans, 31.7% have hypertension. Among Hispanics or Latinos, 20.6% have hypertension.

Heart:
Among African Americans, 10.2% have heart disease (HD), 6.0% have Chronic heart Disease (CHD).
Among Hispanics or Latinos, 8.8% have CHD. circulatory system.

Anatomy of Man	Antiquity Affirmation	Metaphysical Wellness Charge	Physical Disease
I am a shining being. I have been created by and have come into existence from The Most High"	"I speak that I wish to become strong and it comes into being as I speak"	"Arrange for me the ways. May I renew myself. May I become strong."	"Arrange for me the ways. May I renew myself. May I become strong."
Meditate and breathe deeply as you fill your heart with courage.	"I am pure of heart within a pure body. I exist in my heart. May my heart not be taken from me. Let it not be wounded…I know my heart. I have gained power over my heart."	**Metaphysical Dis-ease** Feeling disappointment, unfulfilled, letdown, loneliness, isolation, holding grudges, consumed with fear. **Power Charge** "I have profound courage to live fully. I am forgiven and I forgive."	**Physical Dis-ease** Heart palpitations, heart attack, stroke, clogged arteries
Bloodstream Meditate and breathe deeply as you fill your bloodstream with the light of purification.	"I have made myself whole and sound. I have become young.	**Metaphysical Dis-ease** Deep-rooted generational anger and resentment. **Power Charge** "I am as balanced as the scales of Maat, I am peace, I am calm."	**Physical Dis-ease** High blood pressure, Anemia
Nervous System Meditate and breathe deeply as you fill your nervous system with the light of renewal.	"I have removed my defects, I cut away corruptible matter. Not a member of mine is without Divinity, or wisdom and protects my body entirely. I am light everyday."	**Metaphysical Dis-ease** Fear of the unknown, lacks trusting of self, relationships and environments. **Power Charge** "I am stress free."	**Physical Dis-ease** Stress, anxiety, nervousness
Circulatory System Meditate and breathe deeply as you fill your circulatory system with the light of your renewal.	"My enemy is given to the fire."	**Metaphysical Dis-ease** Stagnated thoughts and actions. **Power Charge** "I flow like a brilliant waterfall."	**Physical Dis-ease** Numbing of face, hands, and feet

Herbal Compound	Nature Balm	Clay Poultice	Zone Massage
"I come into being from unformed matter. I grow into the form of plants."	"An ounce of prevention is worth a pound of cure."	"In the beginning The Most High gave every people a cup of clay and they drank their life." From Proverbs of Digger Indians	"I am the knot within the olive tree."
Bilberry, Hawthorne, Berries, Gingko	Drink 100% or freshly pressed juice with 1-2 lemons and at least 1 quart of distilled water daily	Blend 1 Tbsp of Heal Thyself Rejuvenation Clay with 4oz of 100% Cranberry juice and water and drink. Complete this process daily.	**Face:** Massage the side of each eye. **Hand:** Massage the palm of each hand. **Feet:** Massage the center of the padding of each foot.
Hawthorne Berries, Corn Silk, Burdock	Drink 16oz. of any dark green leafy vegetable (i.e. kale, chard, spinach) Drink 8-12oz of *unsweetened cranberry juice mixed with equal parts of distilled water *Avoid if you have high blood pressure. Substitute with organic apple cider vinegar	Add 1 Tbsp of Heal Thyself Rejuvenation Clay with 8oz distilled water or fresh vegetable of 100% fruit juice.	**Face:** Massage the jawbones for general stimulation. **Hands:** Completely massage each hand.

Chamomile, Hops, Valerian Root Drink herbal tea and bathe in tub with herbs	50 mg of Vitamin B-Complex 3 times daily.	Apply Heal Thyself Rejuvenation Clay to gauze and place over spine and leave on overnight. Take a warm shower in the morning. Complete this process 3 times a week.	**Face:** Massage jawbones for general stimulation. Hands: Completely massage each hand. **Hands:** Completely massage each foot
Dandelion, Gingko, Red Clover Drink herbal tea and take herbal bath	Drink 4-8oz. of *unsweetened cranberry juice with equal part distilled water *Avoid if you have high blood pressure and substitute with organic apple cider vinegar.	Blend 1 Tbsp of Heal Thyself Rejuvenation Clay with 8oz. of distilled water or vegetable juice and drink 3 times a week.	**Face:** Massage jawbones for general stimulation. **Hands:** y massage each foot

FOOD AS MEDICINE

NUTRITION KITCHEN PHARMACY

Level 2 – Intermediate—Vegetarian

Consume only vegetarian foods. Omit all flesh foods (seafood, beef, pork, lamb, turkey, goat, etc.) Fresh vegetables intake includes 50%-75% live food and 50%-25%, steamed to retain as much of the live enzymes and oxygen as possible.

The Lover Man: Week 4   The Communicator Man: Week 5
The Intuitive Man: Week 6

Liquid Breakfast
Kidney/ Liver Flush
Or
Blue & Black Berry Juice w/ 1-2T Green Life Formula
Master Herbal Tea or Woman's Life Tea

Solid Breakfast

Blue Berries w/blended pears sprinkled w/coconut. Blue berries w/blue corn cereal & almond milk

---

Liquid Lunch

Celery 2 stalks, Broccoli, ½ cup Chard ½ cup. Add 1-2T Green Life Formula

---

Solid Lunch

Salad Live Greens

Romaine Lettuce w/shredded broccoli

Steamed Veggies

Zucchini

Protein

T.V.P. Soya Curry Chicken

Liquid Dinner

Wheatgrass 2-4oz or 1-2T Green Life, 12-16oz water

Solid Dinner

Salad

Steamed veggies, whole grain brown rice

Veggie Protein, Black bean soup

Vision Quest Journal Page

Rise | Shine | Listen | Receive | Activate

Week 3 - The Transformation Man of Renewal

_____

_____

_____

_____

_____

_____

_____

_____

_____

_____

_____

_____

_____

_____

_____

_____

_____

_____

_____

_____

_____

_____

_____

The Power To Heal Is Within

THE COMMUNICATION MAN
OF CONNECTIVITY & CREATIVITY
ARIT 5

"I SPEAK
THAT I WISH TO BECOME STRONG
AND I COME INTO EXISTENCE
AS I SPEAK.
I HAVE COMMANDED MY SEAT.
I RULE IT BY MY MOUTH."

The Communication Man has the ability to shape and reshape life, people, environments, places, and things with his words. The Communicator can enter into a body temple and speak dis-ease out and speak wellness into a sick soul. The Communicator Man can ease pain, clear MAD thoughts, realign one's purpose, open the way to those who have lost direction and begin a new pathway all throughout using charge-conscious words that heal.

The Communicator speaks words as medicine and therefore gets you out of harm's way. The Communicator speaks you up from the depths of the Earth and inspires you to grow beyond your apparent limitations. The Communicator said be encouraged and live your life to the fullest and because The Communicator has spoken to you with such strength and conviction, love and understanding, you do.

EMPOWERMENT & DETOX AFFIRMATION
5TH ARIT

May my thyroid center, which houses my throat function in optimal wellness. May I speak myself into wholeness from limb to limb. I now speak words of power, words of strength, words of renewal, words to uplift every body member. May my body, mind and spirit respond with assurance, for my mind and heart are connected to my words and my body is connected to my entire anatomy. My body and my words are one. I send messages of wellness and aliveness to each muscle, nerve, bone, and joint and my body honors the words from my mouth.

WEEK 5 - THE COMMUNICATION MAN OF CONNECTIVITY AND CREATIVITY

The Communication Man dwells in the throat center that houses the lungs and throat.

Statistics: Lungs- -African American men in particular are at risk, they are 37 percent more likely to develop lung cancer than white men http://www. lungusa.org/assets/documents/publications/lung-disease-data/ala-lung-cancer-in-african.pdf

Throat -African American men have the highest incidence of throat cancer (approximately 12 percent)

http://www.mayoclinc.org/throat-cancer/diagnosis.html

Anatomy of Man	Antiquity Affirmation	Metaphysical Wellness Charge	Physical Disease
I am a shining being. I have been created by and have come into existence from The Most High"	"I speak that I wish to become strong and it comes into being as I speak"	"Arrange for me the ways. May I renew myself. May I become strong."	"Arrange for me the ways. May I renew myself. May I become strong."
Lungs Meditate and breathe deeply as you fill your lungs with transformation.	"Grant that I may come forth. May I advance upon the earth."	**Metaphysical Dis-ease** Suppressed and feeling closed in and stifled. **Power Charge** "I breathe fearlessly.	**Physical Dis-ease** Asthma, shortness of breath, emphysema, bronchitis
Throat Meditate and breathe deeply as you fill your throat with the light of conviction.	"I speak that I wish to become strong and I come into existence as I speak. I have com-manded my seat. I rule it by my mouth."	**Metaphysical Dis-ease** Loss of voice, too insecure to speak, fear of rejection. **Power Charge** "I will express my truth."	**Physical Dis-ease** Enlarged thyroid, hypothyroidism, hyper-thyroidism

Herbal Compound	Nature Balm	Clay Poultice	Zone Massage
"I come into being from unformed matter. I grow into the form of plants."	"An ounce of prevention is worth a pound of cure."	"In the beginning The Most High gave every people a cup of clay and they drank their life." From Proverbs of Digger Indians	"I am the knot within the olive tree."
Licorice, Lungworth, Ginger, Mullein	Take 1-2 pieces of leeks, 1-2 cloves of garlic and add to live vegetable or green juice.	Apply Heal Thyself Rejuvenation Clay to gauze and place over the back (where the lungs are located) and leave on overnight. Take a shower in the morning and wash clay from the back. Complete this process at least 3 times a week.	**Face:** Massage above and the sides of the lips. **Hand:** Massage the center of the palm of each hand. **Feet:** Massage above the padding of each foot.
Eucalyptus, Mullein, Motherworth	Seaweeds (dulse, kelp and nori) can be added to salad or vegetable soup. Juice fresh broccoli and brussel sprouts	Apply Heal Thyself Rejuvenation Clay to gauze and place over the throat and leave on overnight. Take a shower in the morning and wash from throat. Complete this process at least 3 times a week.	**Face:** Massage the entire throat area. **Hand:** Massage the middle of the thumb on each hand. **Feet:** Massage the neck of the big toe on each foot.

Vision Quest Journal Page

Rise | Shine | Listen | Receive | Activate

Week 5 - The Communication Man of Connectivity and Creativity

_____

_____

_____

_____

_____

_____

_____

_____

_____

_____

_____

_____

_____

_____

_____

_____

The Power To Heal Is Within

THE INTUITIVE MAN OF CLEAR VISION
ARIT 6

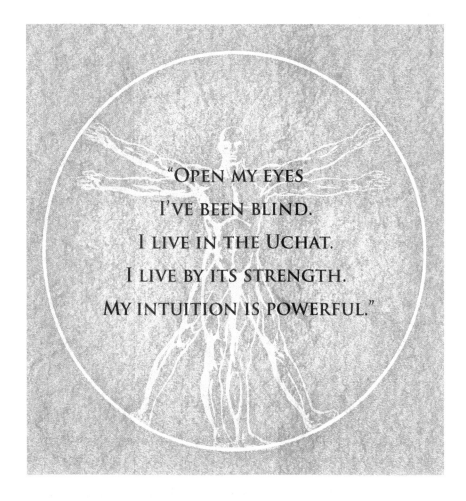

"OPEN MY EYES
I'VE BEEN BLIND.
I LIVE IN THE UCHAT.
I LIVE BY ITS STRENGTH.
MY INTUITION IS POWERFUL."

The Intuitive Man is one who is a seer and who can hear the words from your silent thoughts and interpret them. One who can decipher your past and look clearly into your future. The Intuitive Man trusts himself to be a knower. The Intuitive Man lives in the spirit and by the spirit. The Intuitive Man is connected to his inner voice and that voice carries him through his life's journey. The Intuitive Man feeds his conscious and subconscious mind with inversion exercises, meditation, daily prayer, and green plant foods that strengthen one's intuitive gifts.

PINEAL INTUITIVE EMPOWERMENT AFFIRMATION

6TH ARIT

May my pineal center that houses my intuition, face eyes and mouth function in optimal wellness. May I speak myself into wholeness from limb to limb. May I become a clear messenger of truth. May I receive guidance and protection as I connect to my inner-voice that teaches me moment by moment by moment how to live my life in complete oneness with my purpose. May I listen, trust, act and protect my inner-vision so that I become the greatness that I was born to be. May the serenity in my eyes and the youthful expression in my face, the words from my mouth reflect the oneness in my mind.

WEEK 6 - THE INTUITIVE MAN OF INNER VISION

The Intuitive Man dwells in the indigo pineal energy center that houses the mouth, eyes, and face.

Statistics: Glaucoma is the most common cause of blindness among people of African descent... develop glaucoma early in life, and they tend to have a more aggressive form of the disease. http://www.emedicinehealth.com/primary_open-angle_glaucoma/article_em.htm

Anatomy of Man	Antiquity Affirmation	Metaphysical Wellness Charge	Physical Disease
I am a shining being. I have been created by and have come into existence from The Most High"	"I speak that I wish to become strong and it comes into being as I speak"	"Arrange for me the ways. May I renew myself. May I become strong."	"Arrange for me the ways. May I renew myself. May I become strong."
Eyes Meditate and breathe deeply as you fill your eyes with the light of new beginnings.	"I open my two eyes which have been blind."	**Metaphysical Dis-ease** Inability to see the truth within yourself or others, afraid to see the truth. **Power Charge** "My eyes embrace the truth and I am set free."	**Physical Dis-ease** Heart palpitations, heart attack, stroke, clogged arteries
Face Meditate and breathe deeply as you visualize and fill your face as radiant as a thousand suns.	"My face is of Ra (Sunlight)."	**Metaphysical Dis-ease** Because of the attack on the manhood, one can begin to feel inferior, less than whole, shame-filled, mentally wounded, etc. **Power Charge** "My face reflects the most high within me."	**Physical Dis-ease** Acne, blackheads, age lines, sunken drawn face, swollen face, blotchy skin, sinus infection, etc.
Mouth Meditate and breathe deeply as you fill your mouth with the light of love.	"I am pure from foul emanations."	**Metaphysical Dis-ease** Speaking words of venom and rage. **Power Charge** "I will speak words of healing medicine for I am power-filled."	**Physical Dis-ease** Loose teeth, bleeding gums, tooth discoloration

Herbal Compound	Nature Balm	Clay Poultice	Zone Massage
"I come into being from unformed matter. I grow into the form of plants."	"An ounce of prevention is worth a pound of cure."	"In the beginning The Most High gave every people a cup of clay and they drank their life." From Proverbs of Digger Indians	"I am the knot within the olive tree."
Bilberry, Hawthorrne Berries, Gingko	Drink 100% or freshly pressed juice with 1-2 lemons and at least 1 quart of distilled water daily	Blend 1 Tbsp of Heal Thyself Rejuvenation Clay with 4oz of 100% Cranberry juice and water and drink. Complete this process daily.	**Face:** Gently massage area over the eyelids in a circular motion. **Hand:** Massage the third finger from the pinky on both hands. **Feet:** Massage the first and second toes from the big toe on each foot.
Aloe Vera Gel	Apply alternately warm and cool compresses over the face	Apply Heal Thyself Rejuvenation Clay over the entire face and leave on for 30 minutes, then take a warm shower and wash clay from the face. Apply Aloe Vera Gel after clay is removed from the face. Complete this process at least 3 times a week.	**Face:** Massage the entire face. **Hands:** Massage the tip to the middle of the thumb on each hand. **Feet:** Massage all ten toes.
Dandelion, Alfalfa, Mint, Heal Thyself Breath of Life Formula Drink herbal tea and bathe in tub with herbs	Drink 16 oz. of 100% vegetable juice, ¼ turnip, ½ cup of kale, ½ cup of broccoli, with 1 Tbsp of Heal Thyself Green Life Nutritional Formula	Brush teeth and tongue and massage gums with Heal Thyself Rejuvenation Clay after each meal. Rinse out mouth with warm water.	**Face:** Massage jawbone area on both sides of the face. **Feet:** Massage the neck of the big toe on each foot

Vision Quest Journal Page

Rise | Shine | Listen | Receive | Activate

Week 6 - The Intuitive Man of Inner Vision

_____

_____

_____

_____

_____

_____

_____

_____

_____

_____

_____

_____

_____

_____

_____

_____

_____

_____

_____

_____

_____

_____

_____

The Power To Heal Is Within

THE UNIVERSAL HUMANITARIAN MAN OF GLOBAL WELLNESS

ARIT 7

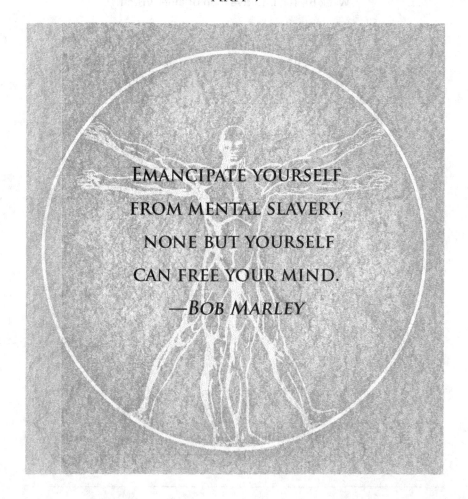

EMANCIPATE YOURSELF
FROM MENTAL SLAVERY,
NONE BUT YOURSELF
CAN FREE YOUR MIND.
—BOB MARLEY

The Universal Man is in alignment with supreme consciousness with the light, the Source, with NTR, with God, with Olodumare, Allah Jesus, all the many names of the Most High.

The Universal Humanitarian Man contains air, fire, water, earth, the SUN, stars and the moon which flows clockwise- the direction of optimal wellness rather than counter –clockwise flowing in the direction of dis-ease, toxicity, pain, suffering and lack.

The Universal Man is in harmony with the source of life and receives optimal guidance from The Source which gives the Universal Man supreme knowledge.

PITUITARY VISIONARY EMPOWERMENT AFFIRMATION

7TH ARIT

May my pituitary center, which houses my crown, mind, hair, and scalp function in optimal wellness. May my connection with the source of creation assist me in uplifting and unifying humanity into harmony. May the healing of my crown reflect the abundant vitality in my pituitary as my crown reflects the abundant vitality in my pituitary and in my higher consciousness. I will vision myself and all my relations renewed in body, mind, and spirit.

WEEK 7 - THE UNIVERSAL HUMANITARIAN MAN

The Universal Man of Vision dwells in the violet pituitary center that houses the hair/scalp and mind/brain.

Stroke – the incidence of stroke in African-American males is approximately 93 per 100,000, with a death rate of approximately 51 percent. http://www. theuniversityhospital.com/stroke/stats.htm

Anatomy of Man	Antiquity Affirmation	Metaphysical Wellness Charge	Physical Disease
I am a shining being. I have been created by and have come into existence from The Most High"	"I speak that I wish to become strong and it comes into being as I speak"	"Arrange for me the ways. May I renew myself. May I become strong."	"Arrange for me the ways. May I renew myself. May I become strong."
Hair Meditate deeply as you fill your hair and scalp with the light of promise	"My hair is of Nu (Primordial water)."	**Metaphysical Dis-ease** Weak, fatigue and stressed state of being. **Power Charge** "My hair and scalp are vibrant. I am alive and crowned in well-being."	**Physical Dis-ease** Thin, balding, premature graying hair. Dry and dandruff-filled itchy scalp.
Mind Meditate and breathe deeply as you fill your mind with the light of the Most High.	Emancipate yourself from mental slavery, no one but yourself can free your mind." –Bob Marley	**Metaphysical Dis-ease** Lack of vision. Mentally "stuck in a rut". **Power Charge** "My mind is powerful, centered and charged. I am alert, clear and in tune. I am mentally fortified."	**Physical Dis-ease** Poor memory, headaches, depression, insomnia, stroke, cardiac arrest

Herbal Compound	Nature Balm	Clay Poultice	Zone Massage
"I come into being from unformed matter. I grow into the form of plants."	"An ounce of prevention is worth a pound of cure."	"In the beginning The Most High gave every people a cup of clay and they drank their life." From Proverbs of Digger Indians	"I am the knot within the olive tree."
Horsetail, Oat Straw, Nettle, and Alfalfa	Vigorously massage your scalp with Vitamin E (2,500 IU) twice a day.	Apply Heal Thyself Rejuvenation Clay to the scalp, cover with a towel and leave on overnight 3 times a week. Wash clay from scalp in the morning.	**Face:** Massage the forehead and temple areas. **Hand:** Massage the tip of the thumb on each hand. **Feet:** Massage the big toe on each foot.
Herbal Gingko, Gotu Kola	Flaxseed Oil, 30 minute -1 hour *salt baths, sunlight. *Avoid salt if you have high blood pressure. Instead use organic apple cider vinegar	Add 1 Tbsp of Heal Thyself Rejuvenation Clay with 8oz distilled water or fresh vegetable of 100% fruit juice.	**Face:** Massage the forehead and temple areas and across the back of the neck. **Hand:** Massage the tip of the thumb of each hand. **Feet:** Massage the big toe on each foot.

FOOD AS MEDICINE

WEEK 7 NUTRITION KITCHEN PHARMACY

Beginning of 21 Day Live Diet

LEVEL 3 – ADVANCED VEGAN (RAW)

Consume 100% live uncooked food. Live foods include organic live proteins (sprouted beans, raw soaked nuts and seeds, avocadoes), salads, live soups, uncooked grains such as couscous, tabouli, bulgur wheat etc. Consume whole or juiced fresh fruits and vegetables. Drink daily warm water (8oz glasses), 5 cups Master Herbal tea and 8oz of Kidney-Liver Flush.

Liquid Breakfast
Kidney/Liver Flush
8oz. Unsweetened Cranberry Juice w/1-2 T Green Life
*Master Herbal Tea or Woman's Life Tea**
Solid Breakfast
Diced pears w/blueberries strawberries,
or raspberries Blend to a sauce or slice
fruit Pumpkin seed soak ½ cup soaked
pumpkin seeds for the prostate
Liquid Lunch
Blood Restorer ½ cup Kale, ½ cup
chard, 1-2 red radishes, ¼ up ginger
root, ½ beet & 2T Green Life

Solid Lunch

Salad Live Greens: Grated beets & red peppers

Steamed Veggies: 1 cup raw okra with olive oil

& spike sprinkled

Starch: Wrap mock tuna in lettuce or seaweed

wrapped in lettuce or seaweed

Protein: Broccoli sprouts or mung bean

½ cup over mock tuna or salad

Liquid Dinner

Repeat Juice Lunch, add 1-2T Green Life

Solid Dinner

Salad Live Greens: Spinach, mung bean & soaked

Steamed Veggies: Steamed or live okra

Starch: Soaked couscous

Protein: 2T of tamari in sauce over grain

or ½ avocado

Vision Quest Journal Page

Rise | Shine | Listen | Receive | Activate

Week 7 - The Universal Humanitarian Man

_____

_____

_____

_____

_____

_____

_____

_____

_____

_____

_____

_____

_____

_____

_____

_____

_____

The Power To Heal Is Within

CHAPTER 6

THE JOURNEY TO BECOMING THE SUPREME MAN OF OPTIMAL WELLNESS

THE LAST 5 ARIT STATES OF MAN (8 -12)

Arit State 8:
The Illuminated Man of Enlightenment

Arit State 9:
Harmonizing Man of Serenity

Arit State 10:
The Nature Man of Regeneration

Arit State 11:
The Alchemist Man of Change

Arit State 12:
The Supreme Man of Optimal Wellness

"THE FUTURE OFFERS EACH OF US
SIGNIFICANT CHALLENGES AND
OPPORTUNITIES.

WE CAN REPEAT OUR PAST EXPERIENCES
OR WE CAN EXPLORE NEW LEVELS
OF AWARENESS.

WE CAN CHART A FLIGHT PLAN
FOR SUCCESS".

BOB LAW, CHAIR OF MILLION MAN MARCH, NY COMMITTEE

JOURNEY TO A SUPREME MAN
OF OPTIMAL WELLNESS

Bob Law, who stands 6 feet 5 inches tall, is a Supreme Man. He is one of my heroes. With his calm persona and velvet voice on WWRL air waves he lifted up our community. His profound intelligence and huge heart combined with a careful approach to healing our social dilemmas with his wisdom, made him, not only my hero, but our hero. He loves us.

It was Bob Law who encouraged me to write my first book, the little Green Book, *Heal Thyself for Health and Longevity.* For years, I had really wanted an opportunity to be on his radio show. Then it happened. His vibrant and beautiful wife Muntu Law came to me for a holistic consultation. Muntu Law and I bonded. She said her husband could also benefit from wellness support. She made an appointment for husband to come and see me.

Once we met and he became familiar with my holistic work, Bob Law blessed me with the opportunity to be a guest on his radio show. That was the beginning of the expansion of my work in a very public way. He fully supported "liberation through purification," the concept I promote as heart of Healing Thyself. I became a regular on his show. In 2000 I was introduced to his "circle", which gave me the opportunity to travel with them to retreats and seminars around the country promoting our shared vision of Wellness. We even went on Wellness cruises.

In 2008, Bob Law held a Wellness seminar for Black Men and those who love them. The panel of presenters included Dr. James McIntosh, Bob Law himself, his wife, Muntu Law, and me, your sister, Queen Afua. Bob Law put out an urgent call around the issue of Black men's health. He presented statistics from the New York City Department of Health that reported that African American consistently had the highest rates of disease in almost all categories. The data covered Black populations in all the boroughs of New York City. Bob Law further stated that as we enter the 21st Century, far too many Black men are dying in their late fifties and early sixties. All too often we are losing our men to poor health care, poor nutrition and poor stress management.

Then Bob Law said, "After a decade of nurturing women, Queen Afua is fulfilling a promise she made in 1995, at the time of the Million Man March. She is turning her attention to the wellness of Black Men". He gave wellness a "shout out" as he told everybody that he had discovered a new strategy to achieve optimal health. He invited the men at the seminar to do the same. He told them what I had been saying about learning to live with Wellness, instead of with avoidable pain. He told them they could learn how to protect their prostate and to cleanse their colon. They could overcome stress and get their blood pressure and diabetic conditions under control.

Bob Law, my brother, kept me close to him while he nurtured me in the process of bringing Wellness to my brothers and sisters. He compelled me to produce my Wellness formulas and make them available to a larger audience. At he seminar Bob Law said to me, "Stick with me kid, I'll help you reach the people with your Heal Thyself mission."

After serving the community and our people nationwide, for three decades, Bob Law has retired from Talk Radio. He is greatly missed. I don't see Mr. Law often now, but he will forever be a part of my work. I recognize him as a Supreme Man because of his commitment of helping me to grow my vision and restore our people to wholeness. During the 1960s and 1970s, Bob Law believed that our right to wellness was a critical part of the Civil Rights Movement. He was then, and continues to be an activist for wellness.

The following segment of Man Heal Thyself takes you on the quest to awaken the Super Powerful, Super Brilliant you. Tap into a holistic, high frequency of living as you evolve to an Illuminated, Man of Balance. Nurture the Nature Man within as you learn to commune with nature. Become the Alchemist Man who transforms himself and others from a deadly lifestyle to a lifestyle of Wellness. Claim your joy and prosperity as you become Supreme Man of Optimal Wellness.

THE ILLUMINATED MAN

ARIT 8

"KEEP YOUR HEAD TO THE SKY..." EARTH, WIND AND FIRE."

The Illuminated Man who releases his past karma and shai trauma and is thus, not a slave to his past life. One who has elevated from toxic karmic-debt.

AS A SUPREME MAN OF RADIANCE, I SIT ON MY INNER THRONE OF ILLUMINATING LIGHT

The Illuminated Man is a Man that shines from within. The Illuminator is a Man who can see the light at the beginning, middle, and end of the tunnel and is able to help you, the seeker of truth, to see the light as well.

The Illuminated Man can make all things possible through prayer, meditation, affirmations, and visualization. The Illuminated Man has risen above jealousy, rage, inferiority, domination, oppression etc. The Illuminated Man has learned from his life lessons. The Illuminated Man is compassionate, loving, and merciful. The Illuminated Man has forgiven himself and all others for their past mistakes and misgivings for he has acquired the blessings, knowledge, insights, realizations, and remedies from his lessons of life and has overcome.

The Illuminated Man has broken toxic habits and patterns that have been created from karmic-debt. The Illuminated Man does not place blame, he takes full responsibility for what he attacks and he takes each opportunity to grow, expand, and learn from his life experiences.

The Illuminated Man is in the world but not of the world. The Nile Valley affirmation of The Illuminated Man: I am that I am, a shining being dwelling in light.

THE HARMONIZING MAN OF SERENITY
ARIT 9

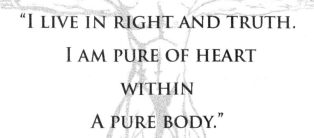

"I LIVE IN RIGHT AND TRUTH.

I AM PURE OF HEART

WITHIN

A PURE BODY."

AS A SUPREME MAN OF BALANCE,
I SIT ON MY INNER THRONE OF HARMONY

The Harmonizer Man is in Supreme Harmony with humanity.

He is one who is able to evoke harmony with his fellow humans, both man and woman.

The Harmony Man is harmoniously connected to his body, mind, and soul. He emanates harmony with family, friends, community, co-workers and all of his relations. As a result, when those who are stressed, or confused come into the presence of The Harmony Man, they are inspired, influenced, and charged to come into harmony.

The Ancient Afrakan term for harmony is Maát.

Maát represents balance, truth, righteousness, and reciprocity.

The Harmony Man's heart is as light as a feather.

The symbol of Maát is the feather.

The ancient Afrakan Nile Valley Civilization was developed on
the Principle of MAÁT.

Maát represented social justice and all on the land had
a natural birthright to Maát (harmony/balance).

FOOD AS MEDICINE

WEEK 10 NUTRITION KITCHEN PHARMACY

LEVEL 4 – ADVANCED WHOLE FOOD THERAPEUTIC JUICE FAST*

Arit & Week 10-11-12

Consume 100% organic liquid meals only. This cleanse consists of two vegetable juice meals for rejuvenation and one fruit juice meal for detoxification, daily. Additionally, there is a daily intake of ½ gallon warm water (8oz. glasses), 5 cups Master Herbal tea and 8 oz of Kidney-Liver flush every day.

Liquid Breakfast
8oz. Unsweetened Cranberry Juice-12oz. w/1-2 T Green Life
(Master Herbal Tea or Woman's Life
Liquid Lunch
Wheatgrass 2-4oz w/ 12-16oz. distilled water or
Beets ½ cup; Kale ½ cup; chard ½ cup 1-2 T Green Life
Liquid Dinner
Spinach ¼ cup or 1-2T Green Life
In 12-16oz pure Water

*Level 4 is a therapeutic juice fast that should be followed for seven days each season (84 days). Elements of the Juice Fast are part of all four steps

THE NATURE MAN OF REGENERATION
ARIT 10

"GOLDEN ARE MY LIMBS,

BLUE MY CROWN,

EMERALD MY BODY."

The Nature Man is in alignment with the harmonic clockwise flow of the Universe and with the flow of Wellness, wholeness, and harmony. The Nature Man knows how to engage with the natural elements and therefore can use air, fire, water and earth to restore, rejuvenate, rebuild and detoxify self and others from mental, physical, emotional and social dis-ease. He lives harmoniously and has reverence for the healing calm of nature.

AS A SUPREME MAN OF NATURE I SIT ON MY INNER THRONE OF NATURAL LIVING

The Nature Man is in tune with the application of:

Earth: Earth foods, vegetables, herbs, fruits, clay, sand and soil

Water: Water foods (cucumber, watercress and parsley);
waterfalls, lakes, rivers and oceans, rain and warm water compresses

Air: Air foods (leeks, scallions and onions), breathing, raw live foods; wind

Fire: Fire foods, sunlight, hot baths and steams and hot springs.

The Nature Man keeps his arsenal of nature tools to use in his healing work.

The Nature Man addresses all concerns and challenges with elements in nature.

The Nature Man has connected that God, Spirit, The One Most High, NTR, Allah

He is within nature and nature is within his High Supreme Consciousness

The Nature Man trusts in nature we have the opportunity to drink,

 bathe, wash, eat, and consume the life force of Divinity.

Nature Man lives according to nature.

He is one with nature, and loves a lifestyle that is in harmony with nature.

The Supreme Nature Man communicates with Air (wind), Fire (sun), Water (oceans, waterfalls),

and Earth (mountains, grasslands, trees and plants)

Just as George Washington Carver, Master botanist, communed with plants to bring healing to humanity. Man can too.

Just like Imhotep, The Father of Medicine, transformed and healed with the forces of nature. Man too, can heal thyself.

THE ALCHEMIST MAN OF CHANGE
ARIT 11

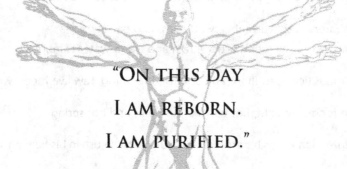

"ON THIS DAY
I AM REBORN.
I AM PURIFIED."

The Alchemist Man has the ability to move and transmute energy in people, places, and things through his thought, word and/or deed.

AS A SUPREME MAN OF POWER I SIT ON MY INNER THRONE OF TRANSFORMATION

The Alchemist Man has developed the gifts of transformation, of mobility, of changing a negative into a positive, of changing toxicity to purity, of changing a challenge into an opportunity. The Alchemist possesses the power of transforming one from a dis-eased state to a state of Wellness, of changing a dark and gloomy situation into a beautiful day, of changing a defeated person into an inspired soul. The Alchemist moves energy, people, environments and states of being, to higher ground. The Alchemist Man moves beyond fear and impossibilities. The Alchemist knows that if you can see it in your mind's eye then you can achieve it. The Alchemist Man has the ability to harmoniously influence the physical and energy worlds within and outside of himself. The Alchemist Man is able to transform and transmute energy in people and things because he overstands that he is one with all and just as he can transform himself, he can do so with all things because of he is whole with all things.

THE SUPREME MAN OF OPTIMAL WELLNESS
ARIT 12

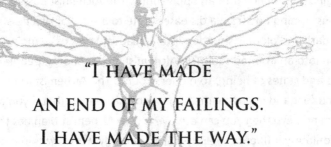

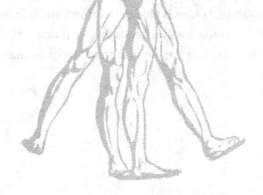

"I HAVE MADE
AN END OF MY FAILINGS.
I HAVE MADE THE WAY."

The Optimalist Man is in Divine Oneness with Source

AS A SUPREME MAN OF WELLNESS, I SIT ON MY INNER THRONE OF OPTIMAL BODY, MIND & SPIRITUAL WHOLENESS

He is the man who actively overcomes his trials and tribulations of pain and suffering. A Man who vibrates and lives to his optimal frequency.

Out of the mud of trials and tribulations, pain and suffering, to the Optimalist Nefer Atum, is a Man who has transformed through the waters of life lessons and has purified himself, thereby has elevated himself out of the mud of Man through the 12 states of Man's inner journey.

The Optimalist Man is the supreme elevated Man. He is totally in oneness and aware of his complete and whole state of being. The Optimalist Man is the Man who rebirthed himself out of the mud of dis-ease, pain and suffering and has therefore liberated himself through purification acts of Wellness. The Optimalist Man is the Man that has blossomed into a Nefer Atum—A Lotus Man of inner and outer beauty. The Optimalist Man has the communication of all 11 Arit from 1-11.

The Optimalist Man is in Divine oneness with Supreme consciousness and he is living the highest frequency known to Man. Through The Optimalist Man's awakening, the world is restored.

PARADISE

What will Paradise be for The Supreme Man of Optimal Wellness?

In the Islamic faith, it is said that if a man lives a righteous Muslim life when he goes to the afterworld he will enter into paradise and have beautiful virgins as his reward. Before his transition, world-renowned Supreme Historian, John Henrik Clarke used to say, "…Paradise is between a black woman's thighs." As The Velvet Sword, I say to this you, Supreme Man of Optimal Wellness, "You have come into your higher self and reflect the God in you. You reflect Neter, Jah, Allah, Jehovah, Krishna, Yahweh, Jesus, Olodumare. And, so, the more you purify your body, mind and spirit, the more you will attract unto yourself a woman who embodies paradise within herself."

It is true that some men attempt to experience paradise with a woman, while they themselves are not living a holistic life. On the other hand, if a man is a seeker of true paradise he will strive to elevate himself beyond the Wounded Man and use his inner strength to become a Wellness Warrior. Courageously, he will continue his quest to become The Supreme Man of Optimal Wellness. His Wellness will be his first reward of many.

You, Supreme Man of Wellness, should look forward to meeting, face to face, a Sacred Woman, a Purified woman, a Mystic woman, a radiant whole woman. She will be someone who shares with you: peace, not war; joy, not pain; balance, not revenge and beauty instead of the ugliness in life. She will be sweet to taste, and lovely to touch, and will emanate a most divine aroma from her body and essence from her spirit.

This Woman of Paradise --your inner vision of delight-- will spring from the garden of your mind and spirit and heart. You will share with each other luscious and tasty vegan foods, greens, herbs, live juices and pure water. She is free from physical dis-ease and emotional toxicity. Your bliss will shine in and from your relationship, like a million shining stars because together you create and share a fulfilling lifestyle. This Woman of Paradise is energetic and wise and radiant. You share the path of wellness and area a divine reflection of consciousness and each other. You meet in the Paradise that you have each created from within. Together you will conceive and birth a new world of Divine Order; of Paradise on earth. Heaven.

Vision Quest Journal Page

Rise | Shine | Listen | Receive | Activate

Week 8 - The Illuminated Man of Enlightenment

_____

_____

_____

_____

_____

_____

_____

_____

_____

_____

_____

_____

_____

_____

_____

_____

_____

_____

_____

_____

_____

_____

_____

The Power To Heal Is Within

Vision Quest Journal Page

Rise | Shine | Listen | Receive | Activate

Week 9 - The Harmonizing Man of Serenity

_____

_____

_____

_____

_____

_____

_____

_____

_____

_____

_____

_____

_____

_____

_____

_____

_____

_____

The Power To Heal Is Within

Vision Quest Journal Page

Rise | Shine | Listen | Receive | Activate

Week 10 - The Nature Man of Regeneration

_____

_____

_____

_____

_____

_____

_____

_____

_____

_____

_____

_____

_____

_____

_____

_____

_____

_____

_____

_____

The Power To Heal Is Within

Vision Quest Journal Page

Rise | Shine | Listen | Receive | Activate

Week 11 - The Alchemist Man of Change

_____

_____

_____

_____

_____

_____

_____

_____

_____

_____

_____

_____

_____

_____

_____

_____

_____

The Power To Heal Is Within

Vision Quest Journal Page

Rise | Shine | Listen | Receive | Activate

Week 12 - The Supreme Man of Optimal Wellness

The Power To Heal Is Within

CHAPTER 7

FINAL
THOUGHTS

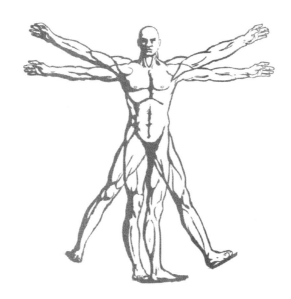

CHANGE

When you could not see yourself…beyond your imperfections and short comings, I saw you…your greatness… your radiant beauty… I knew you would overcome, make it happen…

Man, Heal Thyself. Your roots are your family members and those who came before you. All that you are has been passed down to you – sperm to ovum – man to woman – generation to generation. The seeds they planted yesterday -- peace, war, wellness, madness, strife, serenity-- represent their love denied and their love realized. Those seeds are in you. You are the sum total of what was planted into your bloodline.

Man, Heal Thyself. You do not have to remain a prisoner of the negative elements in your DNA, such as, mother's diabetes, father's prostrate cancer, grandfather's Alzheimer's disease, or grandmother's fears. If you make changes to your lifestyle, you, and your future bloodline can enjoy peace and Wellness. You can restore your Spiritual Wellness through prayer and mediation. You can detox from dis-eases and purify your physical anatomy by eating "live" foods, doing your body work and striving to live a more holistic lifestyle. You can look at how you eat and how you live and decide what is working for you and what needs to be changed.

Man, pick up your bag and start walking on your twelve week journey to Optimal Wellness. With determination and commitment you can rejuvenate your total being –physical, mental, spiritual, emotional, social and even financial. You can overcome the negative DNA. As you holistically transform into a Heal Thyself Man you will be planting new seeds for the next generations. Your life and the lives of your future family will be restored. Many have gone before you planting good seeds and doing good work. Now it is your time. As a human you have a birthright to wellness. As a Heal Thyself Man, you have a responsibility to make your wellness happen. Make that change.

QUEEN AFUA

I'm starting with the man in the mirror

I'm asking him to change his ways

And no message could have been
any clearer

If you wanna make the world
a better place

Take a look at yourself
and then make a change

Michael Jackson
August 29th, 1958 - June 25, 2009

(Man Heal Thyself Thanks You, MJ, a global, healing visionary. All praises.)

GLOSSARY

1. **Arit** - energy centers (also known as chakras)

2. **Ankh** – ancient Khametic symbol; "Key of Life"

3. **Balance** -- stable, even; (opposite of Imbalance)

4. **Bes** – ancient Khametic deity; protector

5. **Bloodline** – family background; lineage

6. **Clay** – earth; mud

7. **Detox** – (detoxification) - to cleanse from poisons, to purify

8. **African Diaspora** – worldwide involuntary and voluntary movement of African peoples and their descendants

9. **Elements** – basics; Air, Fire, Water, Earth

10. **Flexitarian** – eats mostly vegetables but also some flesh foods

11. **Herbs** – plants used for cooking and/or medicinal purposes

12. **Holistic** – approach beyond just physical; includes mental, spiritual, social etc.

13. **Juice Fast** – meal plan consisting of organic juices and purified water

14. **Khamet** – Afrakan term for Nile Valley region (also spelled – Kemet, Khamit)

15. **Principle of Maat** – ancient Nile Valley laws of justice and order

16. **Metaphysical** – refers to non-physical part of the whole person

17. **Million Man March** – African American men gathered for unity and atonement on Oct. 16, 1995, in Washington, DC

18. **Rejuvenation** – restoration; renewal

19. **Toxic Lifestyle** – lifestyle that does not support wellness

20. **Vegan** – eats Live food; eats no flesh foods

REFERENCE AND CITATION SOURCES

Albertine, Kurt H., Anatomica's Body Atlas, Thunder Bay Press, 2006

Alexander, Michelle. The new Jim Crow : mass incarceration in the age of colorblindness.New YorK: New Press, 2010

American Heart Association, Heart Disease and Stroke Statistics: A Report From the 2010 National Survey on Drug Use and Health. September, 2010. Web. 21 December 2011.

Balch, Phyliss, A, Prescription for Herbal Healing, Avery Trade, 2002

Balch, Phyliss, A and James F. Balch, Prescription for Nutritional Healing

Avery Trade, 2010

Budge, E. A. Wallis. THE PAPYRUS OF ANI (THE EGYPTIAN BOOK OF THE DEAD), 1913, New York: Putnam

Dale, Cyndi, The Subtle Body: An Encyclopedia of Your Energetic Anatomy, Sounds True, Colorado, 2009

Gerber, Richard. PRACTICAL GUIDE TO VIBRATIONAL MEDICINE: Energy Healing & Spiritual Transformation, New York: Harper-Collins, 2001

Souls of Black Men: African American Men Discuss Mental Health, Community Voices, Satcher Health Leadership Institute of Morehouse School of Medicine. 21 July, 2003, Web: 21 December 2011.

Stone, Robin, D. No Secrets No Lies: How Black Families Can Heal from Sexual Abuse, Robin D. Stone, Broadway, 2004.

Substance Abuse and Mental Health Services Administration. (2011). "Results from the 2010 National Survey on Drug Use and Health: Volume I. Summary of National Findings" Web: 6 Jan, 2012

Udo, Erasmus. "Fats That Heal, Fats That Kill: The Complete Guide to Fats, Oils, Cholesterol and Human Health". Alive Books, 1993

ACKNOWLEDGMENTS

I am grateful for *uncountable blessings* from on **High.**

To the Ancestors:
"I acknowledge all the ancestral Holistic Healing Men whose shoulders I stand upon to continue the Wellness Work. Special gratitude to Wellness Warriors: Imhotep of the Nile Valley, Father of Ancient and Modern Medicine and Dr. George Washington Carver, Genius Botanist and Herbalist. To my Giant of a Father, Ephriam Robinson, Grand Exalted Ruler and entrepreneur, you adored me. Thank you, Daddy, for nourishing your daughter, Helen, at our kitchen table chats. You gave me the words of Honorable Marcus Garvey and taught me to believe in myself, even if in the line fire. To Dr. John E. Moore, Master Herbalist, for believing in my healing vision quest. To talented teachers Baba Kwame Ishangi, master dancer/musician and Baba Olatunji, master percussionist/vocalist for over four decades. To Dr. Ronald Davidson, an ancestor too soon, you lived the union of allopathic and holistic healing long before it was fashionable."

Profound gratitude to: "To my Sons, Supa Nova Slom and Ali, for being my original Wellness Warriors. To my granddaughter, Atnnt, for recognizing that half a man is one *on his way* to MAN HEAL THYSELF. To daughter Sherease, my heart."

I am grateful for beloved elders, activists, entrepreneurs and inspirations; each in your own way, Wellness Warriors: "I give thanks to Sen Ur Ankh Ra Semahj Se Ptah (The Studio of Ptah) for masterfully teaching the wisdom of the Nile Valley Legacy; to Bob and Muntu Law for years of leadership, encouragement and support; to pioneers and herbalists Dr. Llaila O. Afrika, Dr. Sebi, and Dr. Paul Goss, for your life-long dedication. To Jesse Brown, master colon therapist, in Detroit and the Mud Man of Philly, each for spreading the word. Brother Wanique Shabazz, for sounding the radio "drum" in Atlanta and Imhotep Gary Byrd, for keeping the community informed on the Gary Byrd Experience. To Barack Obama for wanting to encourage wellness programs. I look forward to that vision coming to pass. Sofia Bandele, former Director of the Medgar Evers Women's Center, you are a fearless warrior; Pastor Johnny Ray Youngblood, you are a fearless pastor. Frederica Bey, daughter Amina and the good souls at WISOMMM your generosity was a blessing."

Thank you for music and dance and beauty:
"Katriel Wise and wife, Empress Thandi for being the essence of Wellness ,music and beauty; Abdel Salaam and wife, Dyane Harvey-Salaam for founding Forces of

Nature; and Ben Vereen; Dead Prez; Common; Stevie Wonder, Erykah Badu, for your healing artistic talents. Baba Obediah Wright, director/ choreographer/actor, thank you, for teaching me. Ralph Carter, thank you for your songs and laughter. Orajay, you are the Beauty Shaman."

Gratitude to: "Clement Toussaint, at eighty, you are a vibrant symbol of Man Heal Thyself. Thanks Etta Dixon, you are a Dancing Senior and a Mother of Heal Thyself Purification. Gratitude, Attorney Kenneth Hagood, Honorable Hannibal Ahmed, and Brother Enrique Colon, for following your spirit and becoming the first official "graduates" of Man Heal Thyself training. To Baye Sif Mudti Yanu, you naturally walk the path of a Supreme Man. To King Simon and Brother Polite and Tunde Re and TaharQaka Aleem gratitude for all your Wellness Work. Sacred Woman Soul Sweat Society, for detoxing with me each month as my vision for Man Heal Thyself became clearer; thank you for the company. To all the men who taught me about Men. To Nubian sons ,including Kuji, Inter-Fy , Lou Quantum Leap, Kazi, Kufu, Omni, Phoenix, Rafi and Revolution. I love the Warriors you are."

Blessing and thanksgiving for the birthing of this book: "Supa Nova and Ali, you would not let me not write Man Heal Thyself. Sister from another mother, Dr. Bernadette Sheridan, you continue to be a brilliant , dedicated believer in the union of allopathic and holistic. Dianna Pharr and Lady Prema, for supporting my life's work. To Errol Richards, for your vision of the Master Healers Tour. To Erykah Badu and Big Mike and Attorney Ward White for taking the Walk of Faith to launch *Man Heal Thyself.* Tito, your artistic talent brought the heart of the Arit men to the book. Cindy Shaw, once again your skills and your patience are invaluable. Autumn, thank you for typing and research. Dear staff, Dr. Seshatms Maatnefert, Nivia Goldson, Andrea Spencer, thank you for keeping the center running smoothly, and my devoted, typing team for struggling - with grace- through my handwriting. Dawn Walton you brilliantly and tenaciously "dotted i's and crossed t's ." To Joan Adams for your generosity in the form of research skills. And, last but not least, Gerianne Scott, Midnight Literary Midwife, you have been on this ride with me since my first book, over a quarter of a century ago; you are still here. Salute. I love you for understanding my visions."

Profound gratitude and love to my Mother, Ida Robinson. "Thank you for being the vigilant guardian of my life and my work."

QUEEN AFUA

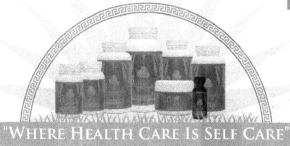

"WHERE HEALTH CARE IS SELF CARE"

The 21 day Detox Program has been clinically proven to enhance wellness. Queen Afua has laid out the "greenprint" to transforming your health in 21 Days. In the 21 Day/ 4 module detoxifying regimen, you will learn how to slow down the aging process, lose weight, and gain optimal health and vitality. Rejuvenate with food as medicine, wellness formulas and consultations to help overcome diabetes, heart diseases, fibroids, prostate blockage, obesity, fatigue and stress. Discover how to achieve peace and well-being in your home and in your life for health, beauty and longevity.

ORDER NOW MAN HEAL THYSELF 21 DAY DETOX KIT
PROGRAM INCLUDES:

Green Life Nutritional Formula -
Builds the immune system and helps eliminate excessive hunger.

Master Herbal Detox Formula -
Purifies and restores all of the bodily organs. Cleanses the bloodstream, rejuvenates the brain, lungs and bones.

Colon Ease Formula -
Lubricates the colon to ease elimination of old impacted waste from the large and small intestines.

Herbal Laxative Formula -
Gently draws 1-2 Lbs of impacted waste out of the colon on a daily basis.

Rejuvenation Clay -
Nourishes the body/ organs, releases pain and brightens teeth.

Breath of Life Formula -
Assists in alleviating: asthma, sinus and lung congestion, snoring and bad breath.

Man's Life Formula -
helps restore prostate wellness, promotes a healthy immune system, aids in elimination of fluid waste.

Woman's Life Formula -
Supports womb wellness.

Nutrition Kitchen Chart -
Gives you "food as medicine" wellness tools including the amazing libertation menu plan and common kitchen herbs for healing.

8 Pyramids of Wellness Chart -
Demonstrates how to raise up from low frequency toxic food to high frequency health whole food that leads to optimal wellness.

Man Heal Thyself Scroll -
This chart is a guide to holisitcally rejuvente the anatomy of man based on Man Heal Thyself book.

Register now for 21-Day self help, hands on, programs and consultations.
Call: 718-221-HEAL (4325)
Visit: www.queenafua.com

Free Weekly Orientation Workshops! Every Tuesday:
6-7pm City of Wellness citizenship town hall welcome.
7-8pm City of Wellness study group. Bring book to session.
8-9pm Man Heal Thyself hour of power. Bring book to session.
Call (805) 360 -1000   **Code**: 822507#

OTHER BOOKS BY
QUEEN AFUA

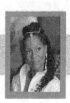

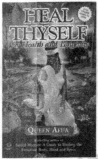

Heal Thyself:
For Health and
Longevity. Guide for
fasting, detoxification
& purification for the
whole family

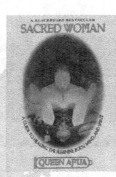

Sacred Woman:
A Guide To Healing
The Feminine Body,
Mind, And Spirit.
Ancient African
lifestyles to awaken
the healer within.

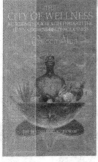

City Of Wellness:
Restoring Your Health
Through The Seven
Kitchens Of Consciousness.
Contains over 250 recipies
to aid the citizens into a
lifestyle of global wellness.

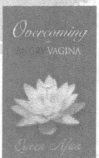

Overcoming an Angry
Vagina:
Journey To Womb
Wellness. Examining the
impact of women's
wellness on overall
wellness around the
globe.

CERTIFICATION PROGRAMS BY
THE QUEEN AFUA WELLNESS INSTITUTE

~ Emerald Green Holistic Practioner Training ~
~ Sacred Woman Womb Wisdom ~
~ Man Heal Thyself Journey to Optimal Wellness ~

For more information visit:
www.queenafua.com
and enroll today!

Selected Titles Published
By
Afrikan World Books

Pale Fox (M. Griaule)..$29.95

Kupigana Ngumi (Shaha Mfundishi Maasi)..$19.95

Yurugu (Marimba Ani)...$29.95

Let The Circle Be Unbroken (Marimba Ani)...$9.95

Melanin: a key to freedom (Richard King)...$16.95

Spiritual Warriors are Healers (Mfundishi Salim)..$29.95

The Isis Papers the keys to the colors (Dr. Frances Cress Welsing)...............$16.95

Blacked Out Through Whitewash (Suzar)..$49.00

Opening To Spirit (Caroline Shola Arewa)...$29.95

Afrikan People and European Holidays vol # 1 (Ishakamusa Barashango)....................$12.95

The Philosophy Of Maat Kemetic-Soulism (Maaxeru Tep)...............................$25.00

The Exhuming Of A Nation (Noble Drew Ali)..$49.95

In The Beginning That Never Began (Almighy God Dawud Allah)...................$10.00

Overcoming an Angry Vagina (Queen Afua)...$20.00

The City Of Wellness (Queen Afua)..$28.00

The Ancient Mysteries of Melchizedek (Melchizedek Y. Lewis)......................$14.95

Over 50,000 Popular & Hard To Find Books

Afrikan World Books
P.O.Box 16447
Baltimore, MD. 21217
Tel# (410) 383 2006
www.afrikanworldbooks.com